Children's Nursing Case Book

Case Book Series

This book is part of a series of case books written for nursing and other allied health profession students. The books are designed to help students link theory and practice and provide an engaging and focused way to learn.

Titles published in this series:

Paramedics: From Street to Emergency Department Case Book
Sarah Fellows and Bob Fellows

Midwifery: Emergencies, Critical Illness and Incidents Case Book
Maureen Raynor, Jayne Marshall and Karen Jackson

Mental Health Nursing Case Book
Edited by Nick Wrycraft

Nursing the Acutely Ill Adult Case Book
Edited by Karen Page and Aiden McKinney

Medicine Management for Nurses Case Book
Edited by Paul Barber

Perioperative Practice Case Book
Edited by Hannah Abbott and Stephen Wordsworth (July 2016)

Children's Nursing Case Book

Edited by Tony Long

Open University Press

Open University Press
McGraw-Hill Education
8th Floor
338 Euston Road
London
NW1 3BH

email: enquiries@openup.co.uk
world wide web: www.openup.co.uk

and Two Penn Plaza, New York, NY 10121-2289, USA

First published 2016

A catalogue record of this book is available from the British Library

ISBN-13: 978-0-33-526462-9
ISBN-10: 0-33-526462-X
eISBN: 978-0-33-526463-6

Library of Congress Cataloging-in-Publication Data
CIP data applied for

Typeset by Transforma Pvt. Ltd., Chennai, India
Printed and bound by CPI Group (UK) Ltd, Croydon, CRO 4YY

Praise for this book

"Developed from a partnership between a University Research Group and an NHS Trust, this practical children's nursing case textbook bridges theory and practice by presenting 23 case scenarios on complex, sensitive and difficult to manage clinical situations in an accessible and user-friendly manner. The inbuilt activities, calculation exercises, question and answer format and extra resources make this an excellent interactive resource for nurses to engage in critical thinking and reflection about each case."

Dr Veronica Lambert, Senior Lecturer Children's Nursing,
Dublin City University, Ireland

"This book will be useful for nurses in the UK who work with children and families in a variety of settings. Its format based on case studies and "what would you do" and "what do you need to do" scenarios will make it a useful tool for teaching clinical care for children and families."

Professor Linda Shields, School of Nursing, Midwifery and Indigenous Health,
Charles Sturt University, Bathurst, Australia

"What Tony Long has achieved is to produce a textbook with contributions from esteemed practicing children's nurses which gives enhanced credibility to each of the case studies. Tony and his colleagues have created these case studies to help children's and young people's nurses fully understand the complexities of the needs of both children and their families or carers during their healthcare trajectory.

The contributors to this textbook fully appreciate that the specificity of knowledge and its application to practice across the parameters of healthcare delivery and across the life course healthcare journey of the child, from the neonatal period through to adolescent transition to adult healthcare, requires a specific knowledge source. This book reflects the reality that children's nurses work in many areas from primary care through to tertiary care, from neonatal intensive care through to child and adolescent mental healthcare. Each of the case studies provides a focal point for this knowledge source and each seeks to illuminate good practice based on sound empirical evidence.

The burden of ill health in childhood can only be alleviated if the nurses who deliver care to children and young people fully understand the complexities of ill health across the age continuum. This is because of what can happen during childhood, from conception onwards, ranging from obesity, heart disease and mental ill health, though to educational attainment and future economic status. Professor Long and his colleagues are to be congratulated in producing this new book which will address each of these cognate areas but which also never forgets the primary mission of the children's nurse which is to uphold their mantra of 'the child first and always'."

Alan Glasper, Emeritus Professor of children's and young people's
nursing at the University of Southampton, UK

Contents

List of figures

List of tables

The partnership of authors

This case book has been produced in partnership between the CYP@Salford research group in the University of Salford and clinical colleagues from Central Manchester University Hospitals NHS Trust. Each case was developed by a combination of clinical and academic nurses, drawing on years of clinical experience and insight into the needs of student nurses.

THE UNIVERSITY OF SALFORD

The University of Salford has established a global presence with a turnover of £189 million, 20,000 students and 2,500 academic and support staff. The University has a particularly strong track record of engagement with external organizations through applied research, consultancy and other knowledge transfer activities. Although primarily a teaching and research institution these external interactions are vital in terms of enriching teaching, maintaining its reputation as a 'real world' university and providing gateways to employment for graduates.

CYP@SALFORD

CYP@Salford is a multiprofessional research group that spans health, social care and education and focuses on enhancing services, improving outcomes and evidencing the impacts on children and families. The research group works closely with colleagues in the NHS, local authorities, the third sector and national networks, and maintains research links with international partners in Finland, Norway, the Middle East, the Far East, Europe and Australia. CYP@Salford continues to build on its established reputation for collaboration with children and young people in education and research through a model based on working with young people and the promotion of active citizenship. Students supported by CYP@Salford are integral members of the research group, adding more internationality to its efforts, and exerting positive impacts on children, young people and families. The group's research programmes are listed below.

Safeguarding children

In this programme researchers work with key partners to tackle neglect, child sexual abuse, and the impacts of substance misuse on children.

Outcomes of hospital-focused treatment and care

Research in the programme is designed to improve outcomes in a range of treatment areas, including quality of life for survivors of childhood brain tumours; children and young people attending accident and emergency (A&E) departments; and the effect of making music for and with children in hospital.

Public health in schools

This research adopts social marketing strategies to address young people's risk behaviour in experimenting with drugs and alcohol, unsafe sex, smoking and weapon-carrying; as well as developing resilience in young people to child sexual exploitation.

Mental healthcare for young people

Self-harm, suicide, young carers, the emotional aspects of female genital mutilation and acculturation are some of the issues that are included in this portfolio of research.

Educating the children and young people workforce

In this field researchers both innovate and evidence the impact of developments in educating professionals to work with children and young people, including exploiting the powerful potential of hi-fidelity simulation.

CENTRAL MANCHESTER UNIVERSITY HOSPITALS NHS TRUST (CMFT)

As the leading provider of tertiary and specialist healthcare services in Manchester, the CMFT treats more than a million patients every year. Its specialist hospitals are home to hundreds of world-class clinicians and academic staff committed to finding our patients the best care and treatments. Its vision is to be recognized internationally as leading healthcare; excelling in quality, safety, patient experience, research, innovation and teaching; and dedicated to improving health and well-being for a diverse population.

The Royal Manchester Children's Hospital provides specialist healthcare services for children and young people throughout the north west of England, as well as nationally and internationally. The hospital sees 220,000 patient visits each year across a range of specialties including oncology, haematology, bone marrow transplant, burns, genetics and orthopaedics. With 371 beds it is the largest single-site children's hospital in the UK.

Saint Mary's Hospital was founded in 1790 and, over the years, has successfully developed a wide range of world-class medical services for women, babies and children as well as a comprehensive genetics centre and an internationally recognized teaching and research portfolio. Its leading edge services are tailored both to meet the needs of the local population in Central Manchester and patients with complex medical conditions referred from other areas in the Greater Manchester conurbation, the North West and beyond.

Community health services provide a wide range of community-based health services for adults and children, supporting health and well-being promotion, minor ailments and serious or long-term conditions. It includes the children's community nursing team, health visiting and school health service, in addition to a vast array of specialist services for children with special or complex needs.

Child and adolescent mental health services provide district child and adolescent mental health services in Manchester and Salford, with a range of targeted services, often provided in partnership with other agencies such as the 16–17 team, child and parent service, children with disabilities, emotional health in schools and the looked after children team.

Notes on the editor and contributors

Tony Long is Professor of Child & Family Health and Director of CYP@Salford. After 10 years' experience in child health nursing and intensive care nursing, and 14 years in six posts in nurse education, he joined the University of Salford in 2002. His own research is in two programmes: improving quality of life outcomes for survivors of childhood brain tumour, and enhancing the impact of early intervention in services for neglected children.

Michaela Barnard is a Lecturer in Children and Young People's Nursing. She worked in a tertiary neonatal intensive care unit (NICU) for 15 years and has previously worked for a number of years as a Bereavement Support Sister. She has worked in higher education for ten years and is a Fellow of the Higher Education Academy. Her research interests relate to support needs of parents following bereavement on a NICU.

Jane Benson is a ward manager in an inpatient child and adolescent service called Galaxy House, based at Royal Manchester Children's Hospital. Galaxy House specializes in working with young people with either eating disorders or pervasive arousal withdrawal syndrome.

Fran Binici is a Specialist Practitioner for Children and Young People with Neuromuscular Conditions at Royal Manchester Children's Hospital. She has been a paediatric nurse for 20 years, working predominantly with children with complex health needs in both hospital and community settings. She is the nurse representative on the newly formed North West Adult and Paediatric Neuromuscular Network, and she works in partnership with national charities that contribute to supporting children, young people and families affected by neuromuscular conditions.

Frances Binns is Consultant and Specialist Adviser for Complex Needs, Autism and Learning Disabilities and a WellChild UK Adviser. With Nursing Times, Unite the Union, NHS and Third Sector awards for work to improve services and care for children with autism at the Royal Manchester Children's Hospital, Frances promotes the model nationally and internationally.

Tracey Bloodworth has worked as a Haematology Paediatric Nurse for 31 years at Royal Manchester Children's Hospital, initially focused on oncology and now with non-malignant haematology cases. She takes the lead in sickle cell and transition in the unit.

Julie Bowden has gained experience by working on a general children's ward, in paediatric intensive care and in school nursing since qualifying in 1994 as a Registered Nurse, Child. Julie completed a specialist community public health degree in 2009 and the practice teacher course in 2013. She is currently Team Leader for the immunization and National Child Measurement Programme screening team in school health for Central Manchester Foundation Trust.

Jude Campbell is the team leader and advanced practitioner for paediatric diabetes and cystic fibrosis-related diabetes at Royal Manchester Children's Hospital. She has an MSc in Advanced Practice and is a non-medical prescriber. She is active locally, regionally and nationally on advisory and education boards for diabetes care within paediatrics.

Patric Devitt is Senior Lecturer in Child Health with a clinical background in children's nursing working particularly with children with cancer and their families. He is a member of the steering group of the Royal College of Nursing's Research in Child Health Group. He researches the quality and effectiveness of services for children and families, and also investigates safety issues for children.

Janet Edgar is a Specialist Practitioner for Cystic Fibrosis and team leader at Royal Manchester Children's Hospital. She has been a paediatric nurse for 30 years and has cared for children with cystic fibrosis for the last 25 years both in London and Manchester. She is involved both locally and nationally in developing care for children and their families from diagnosis to transition to adult service.

Celeste Foster is a Senior Lecturer in Child and Adolescent Mental Health. She is a child and adolescent mental health nurse and an adolescent psychodynamic psychotherapist who has worked in child and adolescent mental health services for 20 years. Her main interests are psychoanalytic approaches to working with adolescents in relation to self-harm, complex psychosomatic presentations and developmental trauma.

Janice Grant is Director of Multi-Professional Postgraduate Studies at the University of Salford. She is a children and young people's nurse and member of the autism special interest group at Royal Manchester Children's Hospital. She has a background in applied psychology and is a member of local and national advisory groups on children's issues.

Leyonie Higgins is a Lecturer in Child Health Nursing at the University of Salford, teaching on undergraduate pre-registration and post-qualifying nursing programmes. She has an interest in young people's health, and inequality for students and patients. Her PhD study focuses on resilience in student nurses and how this can be incorporated into pre-registration nursing programmes.

Natalie Hill became the Clinical Educator for Critical Care at Royal Manchester Children's Hospital in 2013. Her clinical career has been in paediatric critical care (neonatal and paediatric intensive care units) and on the burns unit. She holds a BSc in Health Care and PgCert in teaching and learning in higher and professional education. She facilitates the foundation course in paediatric critical care module, and is a paediatric AIMs (acute illness management) and advanced paediatric life support (APLS) instructor.

Rob Kennedy is a children's nurse with over 20 years clinical experience in children's critical care, trauma and burns. He is a university lecturer with a key interest in the impact and health inequalities experienced by children and young people with autism spectrum disorders. He is active locally and nationally delivering burn care education linked to autism spectrum disorder; the focus of his PhD.

Amy Lamb is an Advanced Nurse Practitioner working in the acute setting based between the emergency department and secondary medicine. With 15 years' experience as a paediatric nurse she has a keen interest not only in service development but in developing nursing practice itself. As an independent nurse prescriber with an MSc in Emergency Medicine, Amy works autonomously in her role in the diagnostic assessment, investigation and initiation of treatment for patients.

Jane Roberts is a nurse specialist for home parenteral nutrition and inflammatory bowel disease at Royal Manchester Children's Hospital. She works closely with the gastrointestinal and surgical team to help support patients in hospital and at home. She has a BSc (Hons) and is a non-medical prescriber and clinical examiner.

Sue Rothwell is Matron for Complex and Tertiary Medicine at Royal Manchester Children's Hospital with an interest in quality and enhancing patient experience. Her background is in emergency nursing. She spent 20 years working in both adult and paediatric emergency departments and is an advanced paediatric life support (APLS) instructor.

Trish Smith is the Paediatric Renal Nurse Specialist at Royal Manchester Children's Hospital. Over 25 years she has developed the home-based dialysis service for children in the North West region, training over 400 children and families to manage dialysis at home. With a MSc Nursing, she has collaborated in research exploring the learning and information needs of children and families with chronic kidney disease.

Andrea Stevenson has a BSc (Hons) Nursing, ENB 240 paediatric oncology and counselling certificates. She has worked as a paediatric Macmillan nurse for 22 years, acting as keyworker in caring for children diagnosed with cancer and their families throughout the North West region. Andrea sits on the North West and Greater Manchester paediatric palliative care forums, working to move paediatric palliative care forward.

Lindsay Sykes is a family support specialist practitioner, working across Royal Manchester Children's Hospital and St Mary's Hospital. With over 20 years' experience of bereavement support, she is a member of a small team that supports families in crisis, particularly when a baby or child dies, as well as working as a volunteer counsellor for the Central Manchester University Hospitals NHS Foundation Trust bereavement counselling service.

Louise Weaver-Lowe is Lead Nurse on the newborn intensive care unit at Saint Mary's Hospital, Manchester. She is both a nurse and a midwife. She is a graduate and also holds a MSc in Health Service Management. Louise has worked in neonatal care for over 20 years.

PART 1
Promoting Health

A 5-year-old girl who is clinically obese

Tony Long and Julie Bowden

Case outline

At 5 years and 4 months old, Sophie started school recently. She is happy and enjoys schools, never having had much upset about separation from her parents, and settling in quickly. The teachers and assistants have noted that she enjoys food but eats only normal portions. On routine assessment of all reception class children, she is found to be obese. Her height is 112 cm and her weight is 25.2 kg. Her body mass index (BMI) is calculated at 20.1, and she is plotted to be on the 98th BMI centile. If a child is above the 91st BMI centile they are seen as being of an 'unhealthy weight'.

---

1 **What are body mass index and BMI centile, and how is obesity determined in children?**

A The body mass index (BMI) is the internationally accepted means to quantify the degree to which an individual of a given height is under, above, or close to the weight of others in a population. In effect, it is used as a measure of excessive weight, assumed to be due to a high proportion of fat, and sometimes as a measure of undernourishment. The calculation is made on the basis of the relationship between body weight and height (Figure 1.1).

In adults, waist size is also an important factor since adults may be muscular (and muscle tissue is relatively heavy), resulting in a misleading BMI calculation. However, children do not have such muscle bulk, so waist measurement is not helpful (Dinsdale et al. 2011). However, age is a vital factor, particularly since height, weight and proportion of fat in the body change during different periods of development.

Meaningful understanding of BMI in children relies upon first comparing a child with the population norms for their age and sex for both height and weight (height centile and weight centile) and then plotting these on a BMI centiles chart to show how the individual compares with the population (Scottish Intercollegiate Guidelines Network 2010). Centile charts show the statistical distribution of a measurement across a population. For example, if a child's height were to be on the 10th centile, for every 100 children of comparable age, 10 would be expected to be similar or smaller and 90 would be taller. This allows

$$BMI = \frac{\text{Body weight (Kg)}}{\text{Height (m)}^2}$$

Sophie's weight = 25.2 kg
Sophie's height = 1.12 m

$$BMI = \frac{25.2}{1.12 \times 1.12} = \frac{25.2}{1.254} = 20.1$$

However, of itself, BMI for Sophie is not helpful. Sophie's age = 5 years 4 months

BMI centile
Plotting Sophie's weight and height centiles on the centile chart for girls 2–8 years shows her to be close to the **98th BMI centile**.

Figure 1.1 Calculating body mass index (BMI) and BMI centile

for tracking of a child's weight over time. The result is categorization as underweight, healthy weight, overweight or very overweight (also termed 'clinically obese'). The charts and additional information may be downloaded from the website of the Royal College of Paediatrics and Child Health (2013).

Activity

Practise the calculation and use of the charts with some real data from children whose parents agree to this. Parents are often keen to see the result, as well as to discover their own BMI score – in private.

2 **What is the concern about Sophie being obese at this young age?**

A Childhood obesity is a worldwide problem, prompting the World Health Organization (WHO 2014a) to describe it as 'one of the most serious global public health challenges of the 21st century'. In England in 2012, around 28% of children aged 2 to 15 were overweight or obese (Davies 2014). The prevalence of childhood obesity in England is monitored through the National Child Measurement Programme (NCMP) by Public Health England (2015). Similar data are provided independently in the devolved administrations of Scotland, Wales and Northern Ireland. The latest data (from 2012 to 2013) indicated a decline in the number of overweight and obese children in reception classes, and possibly in year 6 children, too, although the increase in obesity between these two poles of primary school years remained. Obesity almost doubles from starting to finishing primary school (Health and Social Care Information Centre 2013). The burden of the diseases is not spread evenly. The 2012–2013 data showed that nearly 25 per cent of children in year 6 from the most deprived areas were obese, compared with 12 per cent of year 6 children living in the least deprived areas (Davies 2014).

Children who are overweight or obese are more likely than others to continue as obese adults and to suffer from serious diseases including heart disease (hypertension and atherosclerosis) and type 2 diabetes (Juonala et al. 2011), asthma, obstructive sleep apnoea, musculoskeletal problems and some forms of cancer (Davies 2014).

3   **What should form the basis of intervention?**

A   In effect, the task is to establish balance between energy consumed and energy used. This means that the two elements of intervention are improving diet and increasing activity. The Department of Health (2013) details a strategy to respond to the problem of obesity in children (Table 1.1).

4   **Think about what a 5-year-old would like to eat. Try to make two lists – one of foods that Sophie needs to reduce or avoid, and another of foods that she should eat more. Spend some time examining food labels to see how much sugar and fat are in foods that you think should be eaten. Look at the labels for different presentations of the same foodstuff – low-fat or diet versions and 'no-added sugar' items. Measure out what is suggested as a food portion.**

A   You probably found that food labelling is confusing, and that even foods labelled as 'low-fat' can contain almost as much fat as standard products or be loaded with sugar instead. 'No added sugar' can also be misleading, since there may be a high proportion of natural sugar in a product. Food portions used by manufacturers may not coincide with most people's notions of a portion. Moreover, although a fruit salad is nutritious, a very large fruit salad can contain a large proportion of the day's calorie allowance. Having sorted out what is energy dense and what is not, you still have to consider the need for a balanced diet that contains the essential components (carbohydrate, protein, fat), as well as vegetables and fruit. Think about the particular needs of a growing child, and, not least, what children – and Sophie specifically – want to eat. See the eatwell plate (NHS Choices 2014).

5   **Who should be involved, and what should their roles be?**

A   Since the institution of the Healthy Child Programme (Department of Health & Department for Children, Schools and Families 2009), a partnership approach has been taken in preventative and early intervention services for children and young people, focusing on strengths as well as needs, delivered by the primary healthcare team in association with a range of statutory and third sector agencies. Careful consideration must also be applied to the most appropriate environment in which to discuss issues and to provide

Table 1.1 Diet and activity for children over five

Diet	Activity
• Increase the consumption of fruit and vegetables, as well as legumes, whole grains and nuts • Limit energy intake from total fats and shift fat consumption away from saturated fats to unsaturated fats • Limit the intake of sugars	• Be physically active • Engage in moderate to vigorous physical activity for at least 1 hour every day • Include periods of intense, vigorous activity at least 3 days per week (as developmentally appropriate)

Source: Department of Health (2013).

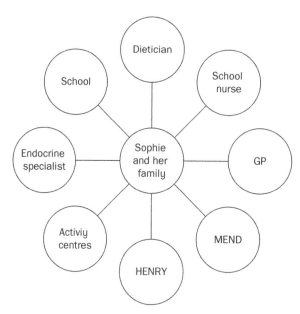

Figure 1.2 The team involved in helping Sophie and her parents

GP, general practitioner; MEND, Mind, Exercise, Nutrition . . . Do it!; HENRY, Health Exercise Nutrition for the Really Young.

supportive interventions. A key issue is to offer support and information rather than to criticize Sophie's parents.

The team involved in addressing the problem for Sophie might include the elements in Figure 1.2. The roles of the nurses, school and third-sector agencies shown in Figure 1.2 will now be considered in more depth. The importance of all such professionals training together to combat obesity has been highlighted by the Royal College of Physicians (2010).

HEALTH VISITOR

Sophie's health visitor works with children up to the age of 4 years and 6 months. She would have carried out a development check at 2 years and 6 months. If there had been concerns then regarding the child's weight the health visitor would have completed an assessment detailing Sophie's diet and exercise, and perhaps asked her parents to complete a food diary. A referral would have been made to a nutritionist, dietician or health lifestyle programme for advice on diet and exercise, and printed or online resources would have been suggested. However, it is clear that Sophie's problem has developed more recently.

SCHOOL NURSE

Following NCMP guidelines, parents are informed, usually by a letter, that there is a concern with Sophie's weight. Once concern is raised that Sophie is of an 'unhealthy weight' her parents can contact the school nurse for further advice. The school nurse can offer them practical advice regarding snack-swapping, portion sizes and means of increasing Sophie's activity. The school nurse would have completed an assessment detailing Sophie's diet and exercise, and perhaps asked her parents to complete a food diary. Referral to the nutritionist or community paediatric dietician will be offered for further advice. If the parents would like more support they can be referred to local healthy lifestyle groups such as MEND (Mind, Exercise, Nutrition . . . Do it, see below). Helpful websites such as Change4Life (www.nhs.uk/change4life) might be promoted. There are regional and local variations, but in one centre, school nurses refer to a dedicated weight management team made up of qualified nutritionists who work with families on changing diet and increasing exercise in home visits. Referral by the school nurse is by parental consent.

GENERAL PRACTITIONER (GP)

In a minority of cases there may be an organic (pathological) cause for the increased weight. This might be an endocrine disorder, for example. Sophie's GP would be informed to initiate referral to a paediatrician or endocrinologist.

SCHOOL

Schools have a requirement to offer at least a minimum amount of two hours of physical education per week in the curriculum. Since Sophie is gregarious, encouraging her to take an active part in physical education (PE) with her friends will help (Table 1.2). Even in reception class, bullying can be a problem, so teachers and assistants will ensure that Sophie does not experience this. Change4Life school sports clubs were introduced by the Department of Health (2013) with the aim of engaging the least active children in sport. Some success has been experienced both in increasing the number of children engaged in competitive sport and introducing physical exercise at a different level for those who were previously inactive. Schools are responsible also for providing healthy options for lunch (Department for Education 2014). Since she has been observed to eat normal portions at lunchtime, Sophie's teacher may review her meal choices and whether additional treats are being provided for Sophie during the school day.

6   **How do non-statutory services play a role?**

A   Many families are more comfortable accessing independent, local services, and this will be encouraged. A wide variety of opportunities are usually available though not always well-publicized. Two examples are detailed here.

HENRY (HEALTH EXERCISE AND NUTRITION FOR THE REALLY YOUNG)

HENRY is a national charity that offers a free service to families with the aim of tackling childhood obesity and promoting a healthy start in life for babies and children (http://www.henry.org.uk/). It also offers training for practitioners in intervening effectively with obese children. As with some other parenting programmes, the intervention is

Table 1.2 The role of schools in responding to childhood obesity

Promoting healthy diets in schools	Promoting physical activity in schools
Help children to make informed choices about food by providing the means for them to acquire life skills and knowledge, and to form positive attitudes and beliefs	Plan curricula to include varied physical education activities every day in order to address different interests and individual needs
Create conditions that promote the adoption of healthy behaviour	Provision of extracurricular sports and activities including non-competitive sport
Increase the availability of healthy food choices in schools	Lead and promote alternative modes of travel to school, ensuring safety but encouraging walking
Ensure that vending machines include healthy choice options as a condition of availability	Develop adequate facilities for physical activity with access for students and the wider community
Raise awareness of the origins of food through school gardens	

Source: World Health Organization (2014b).

founded on principles of solution-focused, whole-family action to provide information about food and activity, with tailored programmes for families to improve parenting skills and confidence, and peer support schemes in the local community.

MEND

MEND stands for 'Mind, Exercise, Nutrition . . . Do it!' MEND 5–7 is a healthy lifestyle programme for 5 to 7 year olds who are overweight or obese (http://www.mendcentral. org/). It involves a programme of weekly sessions of 1 hour and 45 minutes for ten weeks attended by children and their parents or carers. The sessions take place in local facilities such as community centres, schools or leisure centres, and they focus on gradual improvement in diet and physical activity. Activity sessions are supplemented by family workshops and discussion groups for parents. Peer support is a supporting feature. The costs are borne by local authorities and other sponsors.

Activity

Search for comparable local groups where you live or where you work. Think about how you found these, how they can be accessed, and how they seem to be funded. How might families with limited knowledge and perhaps also poor internet access find the opportunities that you identified? Perhaps the role of the primary healthcare team in signposting such services will seem more important.

> **Key points**
>
> - When addressing obesity, serial measurement of BMI is essential for accurate assessment of the problem and of progress.
> - The key to successful management is a combination of controlled calorie intake and increased activity, reinforced with health information and psychological support.
> - A multiprofessional approach is desirable, and schools have a crucial role in providing a healthy diet, encouraging regular physical activity and addressing issues with bullying.

REFERENCES

Davies SC (2014) *Annual Report of the Chief Medical Officer. Surveillance Volume, 2012: On the State of the Public's Health.* London: Department of Health. Available at: https://www.gov.uk/government/uploads/system/uploads/attachment_data/file/298297/cmo-report-2012.pdf (accessed 21 January 2016).

Department of Health (2013) *Improving Children and Young People's Health Outcomes: A System Wide Response.* London: DH. Available at: https://www.gov.uk/government/uploads/system/uploads/attachment_data/file/214928/9328-TSO-2900598-DH-SystemWideResponse.pdf (accessed 21 January 2016).

Department for Education (2014) *School Food in England. Departmental Advice for Governing Bodies.* London: Department of Education. Available at: https://www.gov.uk/government/uploads/system/uploads/attachment_data/file/344684/School_food_in_England-_June_2014-_revised_August_14.pdf (accessed 21 January 2016).

Department of Health & Department for Children, Schools and Families (2009) *Healthy Child Programme: Pregnancy and the First Five Years.* London: DH. Available at: https://www.gov.uk/government/uploads/system/uploads/attachment_data/file/167998/Health_Child_Programme.pdf (accessed 21 January 2016).

Dinsdale H, Ridler C, Ells LJ. (2011) *A Simple Guide to Classifying Body Mass Index in Children.* Oxford: National Obesity Observatory. Available at: http://www.noo.org.uk/uploads/doc/vid_11762_classifyingBMIinchildren.pdf (accessed 9 February 2016).

Health and Social Care Information Centre (2013) *National Child Measurement Programme: England, 2012/13 School Year.* London: HSCIC. Available at: http://www.hscic.gov.uk/catalogue/PUB13115/nati-chil-meas-prog-eng-2012-2013-rep.pdf (accessed 21 January 2016).

Juonala M, Magnussen CG, Berenson GS, et al. (2011) *Childhood adiposity, adult adiposity, and cardiovascular risk factors. New England Journal of Medicine* 365 (20): 1876–1885.

NHS Choices (2014) *The Eatwell Plate.* London: DH. Available at: http://www.nhs.uk/Livewell/Goodfood/Pages/eatwell-plate.aspx (accessed 9 February 2016).

Public Health England (2015) *National Child Measurement Programme Operational Guidance 2015 to 2016.* London: PHE. Available at: https://www.gov.uk/government/uploads/system/uploads/attachment_data/file/463929/NCMP_Operational_Guidance_21015_16.pdf (accessed 21 January 2016).

Royal College of Paediatrics and Child Health (2013) *School Age Charts and Resources.* London: RCPCH. Available at: http://www.rcpch.ac.uk/child-health/research-projects/uk-who-growth-charts/uk-growth-chart-resources-2-18-years/school-age (accessed 21 January 2016).

Royal College of Physicians (2010) *The Training of Health Professionals for the Prevention and Treatment of Overweight and Obesity*. London: RCP.

Scottish Intercollegiate Guidelines Network (2010) *Management of Obesity. Guideline 115*. Edinburgh: SIGN. Available at: http://www.sign.ac.uk/guidelines/fulltext/115/ (accessed 9 February 2016).

World Health Organization (2014a) *Childhood Overweight and Obesity*. Geneva: WHO. Available at: http://www.who.int/dietphysicalactivity/childhood/en/ (accessed 21 January 2016).

World Health Organization (2014b) *Global Strategy on Diet, Physical Activity and Health*. The Role of Schools. Geneva: WHO. Available at http://www.who.int/dietphysicalactivity/childhood_schools/en/ (accessed 21 January 2016).

CASE STUDY 2
A 7-year-old boy who appears to be neglected
Tony Long and Julie Bowden

Case outline

Josh has been doing well at school, appearing to be happy and well cared for. Following the birth of the family's fourth child who has cried excessively since two weeks after birth, Josh's demeanour and presentation have begun to cause concern for his teachers. The school nurse has been asked to review the concerns. The teachers have recorded that Josh is the eldest of four children in the family. Neither parent has been in employment for some years. Josh has started appearing in school in dirty clothes, appearing to be tired and always hungry. He has been seen finishing food left by other children. He has fallen asleep in class on occasions, and his ability in all subjects has deteriorated. The school nurse suspects that Josh is being neglected and that his basic needs are not being met.

---

1 **What is neglect?**

A Neglect is more difficult to define and diagnose than other forms of child abuse. Whereas cigarette burns, for example, are clear to see, neglect can be much less obvious and is often established only when a pattern of signs are observed. Government departments have offered definitions for nurses and social workers to use that reflect this complexity in recognition. The version by HM Government (2015) has been in use for some years now (Figure 2.1). In summary, this indicates that neglect is present when a child's basic needs are not being met, but the range of possible causes is wide. Importantly, neglect may be unintentional.

Neglect is the most common category for child protection registration in the UK (Department for Education 2011). However, neglect can be addressed successfully with skilled, early intervention (Long et al. 2013). Breakdowns of statistics on the incidence of child abuse and different aspects of this are available for different parts of the UK (for example, Department of Health, Social Services, and Public Safety 2012; Welsh Assembly Government 2012).

Efforts have been made to categorize neglect according either to the cause or the effect of neglect (Crittenden 1999, Horwath 2007), and these may help practitioners to order their thoughts about what is usually a complicated set of circumstances and

Definition of neglect

The persistent failure to meet a child's basic physical and/or psychological needs likely to result in the serious impairment of the child's health or development. Neglect may occur during pregnancy as a result of maternal substance misuse. Once a child is born, neglect may involve a parent or carer failing to:

- *Provide adequate food, clothing and shelter (including exclusion from home or abandonment);*
- *Protect a child from physical and emotional harm or danger;*
- *Ensure adequate supervision (including the use of adequate care-givers); or*
- *Ensure access to appropriate medical care or treatment.*

It may also include neglect of, or unresponsiveness to, a child's basic emotional needs.

(HM Government 2015: p. 93)

Figure 2.1 Definition of neglect

Table 2.1 Categorizing neglect

Crittenden (1999)	*Horwath (2007)*
Disorganized neglect	Medical neglect
Emotional neglect	Nutritional neglect
Depressed neglect	Emotional neglect
	Educational neglect
	Physical neglect
	Lack of supervision and guidance

evidence (Table 2.1). Health visitors have been found to recognize both the parental characteristics associated with neglect and the signs in children of developmental problems following such an approach (Daniel et al. 2009).

Increasingly, school nurses are at the forefront of efforts to recognize and address neglect in the school-age years. The Munro report (Department for Education 2011) highlighted the crucial impact of intervening at the earliest opportunity in order to prevent the problem escalating. The Department of Health and the Chief Nursing Officer (2012) identified the vital role of school health services in maintaining and improving the health and well-being of school-aged children, including being pivotal in safeguarding situations. There are well-defined pathways and processes for the school nurse to follow to ensure an effective multi-agency response to Josh's needs.

2   **What might explain the change in Josh's behaviour and appearance?**

A   It is not uncommon for a family to manage well enough until an event occurs that forms a tipping point after which efforts to cope with normal multiple demands simply fail. The stimulus could be the birth of another baby, falling into financial hardship or changes in family composition through one parent leaving, being imprisoned (or released from prison) or entering into a different relationship. Chaotic lifestyles and inadequate care can result. Sometimes it is one particular child who becomes neglected whereas others are relatively well cared for, and the child who suffers may well be the eldest while such parental attention as remains available is directed at the younger children – as in this case.

Josh seems to be showing both physical and psychological responses to the neglect. He is clearly hungry – perhaps missing breakfast or other meals at home, and, therefore, eating whatever he can at school. Being tired at school may be due entirely to this, or it may indicate that he is also losing sleep at home and, perhaps, suffering from a lack of routine. From being previously well-presented he is now wearing dirty clothes, which may mean that he is left to see to his own hygiene needs. All of these issues, however, require more rigorous investigation and assessment.

3   **What will the school nurse do to establish whether Josh is neglected and to promote his well-being?**

A   On receipt of this referral, the school nurse would ask school staff if they had discussed these concerns with the parents. This can be a difficult conversation that some teachers find challenging. Some parents will take on board the concerns that are expressed, and improvements will be seen. However, if, following discussions with his parents, there is no evidence of improvement for Josh, then his parents would be invited to a meeting with the teacher and the school nurse. The purpose of this would be to discuss concerns and to allow the parents to share their difficulties.

The common assessment framework (CAF) will be used to gather information. This is a process used in a standard format across health, social care and education professions to guide efforts to identify a child's needs when a professional has concerns about them and to formulate a plan to ensure that these needs are met. There are four steps in the process: identify the needs (as early as possible); assess the needs focusing on strengths and weaknesses; deliver integrated interventions to meet those identified needs according to an agreed plan; and evaluate the outcomes. All of this is recorded on the CAF form, and parents are an integral part of the planning team. The CAF relies on parents engaging with the process. The focus on early intervention and joined-up working between agencies remains a central pillar of government policy (Department of Health 2013; Public Health England 2015).

Through the CAF process it is possible to establish which agencies should be involved to support the family and ultimately improve the outcomes for Josh. Where appropriate, additional agencies might be invited to attend future meetings, often as additional problems or needs are identified. Referrals should be considered at this stage for further support (perhaps the parents could attend a local parenting group, for example). Ensuring that families are in receipt of the right welfare benefits is a common action.

4   **Think about the problems you might identify and which agencies or services might be able to help with them. Can you think which other professionals might be involved?**

A   The school nurse would liaise with the health visitor who would have had recent contact with this family and may bring a wealth of information regarding the parents' health, housing issues and their financial situation. Agencies need to consider if this family has any support from the extended family and friends. The health visitor would be invited to the next meeting.

The school nurse would also invite parents and Josh to a health assessment at which issues of registration and consultation with a general practitioner (GP), registration and appointments with a dentist, dental hygiene and tooth decay would be reviewed. General health checks may be done at this time, including height, weight, hearing, vision, behaviour, sleep, diet and exercise. Josh's immunization history would be checked. There are a number of resources available to practitioners for such assessments, for example, the Royal College of Paediatrics and Child Health (2013).

Evidence of improvement for Josh should be seen throughout this process. If concerns remain after support is put in place, however, the agencies might consider a joint referral to social services. It would be important to include the CAF assessment and to

---

Principles of good record-keeping (Nursing and Midwifery Council 2010) now encapsulated in The Code (Nursing and Midwifery Council 2015)

The Nursing and Midwifery Council (NMC) states 34 points of guidance regarding record-keeping, including the rules of confidentiality, access and disclosure. Only the first 16 – 'principles of good record keeping' – are reproduced here.

1. Handwriting should be legible.
2. All entries to records should be signed. In the case of written records, the person's name and job title should be printed alongside the first entry.
3. In line with local policy, you should put the date and time on all records. This should be in real time and chronological order, and be as close to the actual time as possible.
4. Your records should be accurate and recorded in such a way that the meaning is clear.
5. Records should be factual and not include unnecessary abbreviations, jargon, meaningless phrases or irrelevant speculation.
6. You should use your professional judgement to decide what is relevant and what should be recorded.
7. You should record details of any assessments and reviews undertaken, and provide clear evidence of the arrangements you have made for future and ongoing care. This should also include details of information given about care and treatment.
8. Records should identify any risks or problems that have arisen and show the action taken to deal with them.
9. You have a duty to communicate fully and effectively with your colleagues, ensuring that they have all the information they need about the people in your care.
10. You must not alter or destroy any records without being authorised to do so.
11. In the unlikely event that you need to alter your own or another healthcare professional's records, you must give your name and job title, and sign and date the original documentation. You should make sure that the alterations you make, and the original record, are clear and auditable.
12. Where appropriate, the person in your care, or their carer, should be involved in the record keeping process.
13. The language that you use should be easily understood by the people in your care.
14. Records should be readable when photocopied or scanned.
15. You should not use coded expressions of sarcasm or humorous abbreviations to describe the people in your care.
16. You should not falsify records.

Figure 2.2 Principles of good record-keeping

Source: Nursing and Midwifery Council 2010: pp 4–5.

provide a detailed account of the support that the family has received so far from the various agencies. Throughout this process, it is important to document clearly the issues, the objective observation undertaken, and the support offered (Beach and Oates, 2014; Nursing and Midwifery Council 2010, 2015, Figure 2.2).

School nursing services also form part of the *Universal Partnership Plus* high-intensity, multi-agency service for children, young people and families where there are child protection or safeguarding concerns (Department and Health and Chief Nursing Officer 2012). For school nurses this means providing a service at four levels with safeguarding being a core part of each level right through from universal services education about protective behaviours, to working as part of a team providing high-intensity services where these are needed.

Key points

- Neglect is a complex issue, and the definition offered in 'Working together to safeguard children' is helpful for all involved to be clear on its potential manifestations and causes.
- Effective multi-agency intervention is achieved through clear communication and agreement about roles. The CAF is central to this.
- Whenever possible, parents are included in discussions about interventions, progress, and possible next steps. This is important since most neglected children continue to live at home with support from health and social care services.

REFERENCES

Beach J, Oates J (2014) Maintaining best practice in record-keeping and documentation. *Nursing Standard* 28(36): 45–50.

Crittenden P (1999) Child neglect: causes and contributors, in H Dubowitz (ed) *Neglected Children: Research, Practice And Policy*. Sage Publications, pp. 47–68.

Daniel B, Taylor J, Scott J (2009) Noticing and helping the neglected child: literature review. London: DCSF.

Department for Education (2011) The *Munro Review of Child Protection: Final Report*. A Child-Centred System. Cm8062. London: Department for Education.

Department of Health (2013) *Improving Children and Young People's Health Outcomes: A System Wide Response*. London: Department of Health. Available at: https://www.gov.uk/government/uploads/system/uploads/attachment_data/file/214928/9328-TSO-2900598-DH-SystemWideResponse.pdf (accessed 16 January 2016).

Department of Health and Chief Nursing Officer (2012) *Getting it Right for Children, Young People and Families. Maximising the Contribution of the School Nursing Team: Vision and Call to Action*. London: Department of Health. Available at: https://www.gov.uk/government/uploads/system/uploads/attachment_data/file/216464/dh_133352.pdf (accessed 16 January 2016).

Department of Health, Social Services, and Public Safety (2012). *Children's Social Care Statistics for Northern Ireland 2011/12*. Belfast: Department of Health, Social Services, and Public Safety.

HM Government (2015) *Working Together to Safeguard Children: A Guide to Inter-Agency Working to Safeguard and Promote the Welfare of Children*. Available at: https://www.gov.uk/government/uploads/system/uploads/attachment_data/file/419595/Working_Together_to_Safeguard_Children.pdf (accessed 16 January 2016).

Horwath J (2007) *Child Neglect: Identification and Assessment*. London: Palgrave/Macmillan.

Long T, Murphy M, Fallon D, et al. (2013) Four-year longitudinal impact evaluation of the Action for Children UK Neglect Project: outcomes for the children, families, Action for Children, and the UK. *Child Abuse and Neglect* 38(8): 1358–1368. Available at: doi.org/10.1016/j.chiabu.2013.10.008 (accessed 16 January 2016).

Nursing and Midwifery Council (2010) *Record Keeping: Guidance for Nurses and Midwives*. London: NMC. Available at: http://www.nipec.hscni.net/Image/SitePDFS/nmcGuidanceRecordKeepingGuidanceforNursesandMidwives.pdf (accessed 16 February 2016).

Nursing and Midwifery Council (2015) *The Code: Professional Standards of Practice and Behaviour for Nurses and Midwives*. London: NMC. Available at: http://www.nmc.org.uk/globalassets/sitedocuments/nmc-publications/revised-new-nmc-code.pdf (accessed 9 February 2016).

Public Health England (2015) *Rapid Review to Update Evidence for the Healthy Child Programme 0–5*. London: PHE. Available at: https://www.gov.uk/government/publications/healthy-child-programme-rapid-review-to-update-evidence (accessed 9 February 2016).

Royal College of Paediatrics and Child Health (2013) *School Age Charts and Resources*. London: Royal College of Paediatrics and Child Health. Available at: http://www.rcpch.ac.uk/child-health/research-projects/uk-who-growth-charts/uk-growth-chart-resources-2-18-years/school-age (accessed 16 January 2016).

Welsh Assembly Government (2012) *Children on Child Protection Register by local Authority Category of Abuse and Age Group*. Cardiff, Welsh Assembly Government.

A 14-year-old girl admitted to hospital after trying alcohol

Tony Long and Julie Bowden

Case outline

Janine was with friends at a party and tried drinking alcohol for the first time. Encouraged by her friends, she drank two 440 ml cans of cider, several shots of flavoured vodka and a long drink of unidentified but certainly alcoholic liquid. She became giddy, then argumentative and finally drowsy although responsive. She vomited once. She was taken to the accident and emergency (A&E) department by a friend's mother. After supportive treatment, neurological assessment and time to recover physically, she was discharged home. The school health team was informed of the episode with the consent of Janine's mother.

1 **Is this a common problem?**

A The problem of teenagers drinking alcohol is improving in England. Surveys for the Health and Social Care Information Centre (2013) show that in 2012 less than half of pupils from 11 to 15 years of age had ever drunk alcohol. This proportion has fallen steadily since 2003. However, the UK generally has far more of a problem than most other European countries (Institute of Alcohol Studies 2013). In the 2012 data, there was a progression in the proportion of pupils who had had an alcoholic drink between 11 years (12%) and 15 years (74%). Behaviour is only one part of the story, though. Attitudes towards alcohol are also important. Drinkaware (2013) reports that 60% of teenagers regard drinking as a normal part of growing up, although most distinguish between trying alcohol and getting drunk.

2 **Why do teenagers start drinking?**

A Curiosity and a desire to fit in with peers were probably the main factors in leading Janine to try alcohol. In time, and through trial and error, most teenagers learn to control their alcohol consumption, although many mistakes may be expected (Percy et al. 2011). Janine is clearly not sufficiently experienced to have developed this state of self-awareness of limits. It was probably not her intention to become drunk, and certainly not to pass out, and her friends may have shared her naivety in encouraging her to drink so much. Percy et al. suggest that becoming too drunk is frowned upon by peers.

3   **What are the risks to Janine of alcohol consumption?**

> ### Extra resource
>
> Try the Drinkaware (2015a) spin the bottle game to see what the risks are and how these relate to Janine's case.
>
> http://www.drinkaware.co.uk/check-the-facts/underagedrinking/the-risks-of-underage-drinking/

A   The amount of alcohol consumed on this occasion is unknown. Uncertainty over what has been drunk (the mystery last drink may have been a cocktail of alcoholic drinks) and how much (unmeasured shots) prevents meaningful control of alcohol intake. Inevitably, this put Janine at risk since she was no longer able to think clearly. Fortunately, she was in a relatively safe environment and with several friends in attendance. Family Lives (2015) reports that more 14 and 15 year olds who drink alcohol engage in sexual activity than those who abstain, and for a significant proportion this leads to unprotected sex.

The World Health Organization (2006) has indicated that there is a direct relationship between the amount of alcohol consumed and likelihood of engaging in violence or serious vandalism. Approximately two-thirds of 10-17 year olds who drink get into an argument and perhaps twenty per cent get into a fight (Family Lives 2015).

School performance can be affected by drinking alcohol frequently since memory and attention are impaired, and many functions of the brain can be damaged either by binge drinking or persistent drinking. Change in personality and social behaviour are possible, and cognitive ability generally can be reduced (Institute of Alcohol Studies 2013).

4   **How will the school health service help Janine and her family?**

A   The hospital would send a copy of the A&E department slip to the school health team, and this will be recorded as part of the chronology at the front of Janine's personal child health record (Royal College of Paediatrics and Child Health 2015). School nurses receiving a one-off A&E slip may not act on this, but if a number of these are presented detailing alcohol-related behaviour then this shows an emerging pattern that will be concerning. The school nurse will then try to speak to the parents to offer advice, as well as speaking to Janine and school staff. Quite often young people will not see the risk involved and will reject any support.

School nurses can meet with Janine to discuss the consequences of drinking too much alcohol. This might take the form of an informal discussion. A health assessment could help to establish whether Janine is at risk of alcohol dependency. She would be directed to websites such as Drinkaware (www.drinkaware.co.uk) for further information. For young people who are alcohol-dependent there are agencies such as Lifeline which can to support young people (http://www.lifeline.org.uk/).

> **Extra resource**
>
> Have a look at the Personal Child Health Record at http://www.healthforallchildren.com/the-pchr/2079-2/. (You will need to enter your name and an email address for copyright purposes.)

SOCIAL MARKETING APPROACH

Some success has been achieved by changing young people's perception of their own risk behaviour compared with that of their peers. In this approach, a survey is conducted asking, for example, 'Have you drunk any alcohol in the last week?'. A follow-up questions asks 'What proportion of others in your year group do you think has done so?'. Invariably, actual engagement in the behaviour (drinking alcohol) is small – perhaps 10 per cent. However, the same individual may believe that 50 per cent or more of their peers drink. Social marketing works by feeding back the positive message that it is normal not to drink alcohol, and that no one should try it just to be like what they wrongly perceive to be the norm. This approach has been used to address smoking, substance misuse, bullying, engaging in sex for the first time or in unsafe sex, carrying weapons and other risk behaviours.

5 **See more about this at http://www.rudifferent.co.uk/. Why might this approach work so well with young people of teen age? In the light of what you decide, think again about Janine's case and see if it alters your thoughts about how such issues should be tackled with someone of her age.**

(A) A POSITIVE CHOICE

It has been argued by young people that adults take the default position of assuming that all young people at least try alcohol when this is not the case in reality (Herring et al. 2012). The young people wanted adults to change the message – to emphasize instead that not drinking at all was a normal and acceptable choice. They denied that drinking and becoming drunk was an automatic rite of passage for young people, declaring instead that those who either do not use alcohol at all or only a little choose to avoid situations in which alcohol will be involved.

In another study, Tucker et al. (2013) found a positive association between media advertisement of alcohol (and other substances) and alcohol usage by teenagers in American schools. Various forms of media exerted differing effects, but the attraction of young people to the many forms of media now in common use risks even greater prompting to try alcohol. Young people may wish to be allowed to remain abstinent, but powerful forces are at work to counter this decision. The role of social marketing in correcting perceptions becomes all the more important in the light of this.

HELPING PARENTS TO TALK TO THEIR CHILDREN ABOUT ALCOHOL

Although the evidence suggests that most children under 17 years of age would ask for information and advice about alcohol from their parents first (Drinkaware 2013), such issues can be especially difficult for parents to address. Even starting the conversation can be a challenge. There is good reason for most parents to be worried about this, since it has been found that most attempts by parents to regulate a teenager's use of alcohol fail to achieve the desired result (Percy et al. 2011). Sometimes, the risk of problems, such as that occurring with Janine, can even be increased by ineffective parental intervention. Fortunately, help is available (although perhaps not often accessed by parents).

Activity

How would you go about speaking to Janine about what has happened and ensuring that further problems are averted? Once you have made a plan and decided what you would say and do, read the tips offered by Family Lives to parents about talking to teenagers about drinking alcohol. The video at the same site on 'Alcohol – don't delay talking about it' is also helpful.

http://www.familylives.org.uk/advice/teenagers/drugs-alcohol/underage-drinking/

Having material for parents to use or share with teenagers is a further helpful way of boosting parents' confidence and effectiveness in talking about alcohol. A variety of these are available. Understanding the law can also help to avoid conflict with the law and to facilitate family occasions (Table 3.1).

Table 3.1 What is the law on alcohol and children in the UK?

	True?	*False?*
Anyone who is aged 16 or over can buy alcohol		
Someone who is 16 or 17 can drink alcohol in licensed premises if accompanied by an adult		
An adult can buy a child over 16 years cider if they are eating a table meal together in licensed premises		
The police can confiscate alcohol from someone under 18 in a public place		
A 5 year old child can drink alcohol at home		
It is illegal to sell alcohol to someone under 18 years		

Extra resource

Once you have tested yourself, check out your answers in the Drinkaware (2015b) leaflet for parents at

http://eb6eac5692db912ed5d9-411b8674dd3ca0f7d171c621142907c5.r53.cf1.rackcdn.com/Parents%20leaflet.pdf

(A slightly different legal rule applies in Scotland [The Scottish Government 2015], in that 16 and 17 year olds are permitted to buy their own beer, wine or cider to drink with a meal.)

Key points

- Before thinking of intervening in a case like this it is vital to take time to understand the context: whether this is an established habit or a one-off foolish decision.
- The best approach is to offer better information and alternative perspectives. Self-directed learning such as exploring website to appreciate the risks involved works well with teenagers.
- Peer pressure and allegiance are of particular importance to teenagers, so social marketing approaches can be especially effective in re-setting perceptions of social norms.

REFERENCES

Drinkaware (2013) *Research into Drinking Attitudes and Behaviour*. London: Drinkaware. Available at: https://www.drinkaware.co.uk/media/157292/drinkaware_attitudes_and_behaviours_executive_summary_2012.pdf (accessed 22 January 2016).

Drinkaware (2015a) *Why Underage Drinking is a Risky Business*. London: Drinkaware. Available at: http://www.drinkaware.co.uk/check-the-facts/underagedrinking/the-risks-of-underage-drinking/ (accessed 21 January 2016).

Drinkaware (2015b) *Your Child or Teenager's Health: Leaflet for Parents*. London: Drinkaware.

Available at: https://www.drinkaware.co.uk/check-the-facts/health-effects-of-alcohol/your-child-or-teenagers-health/your-child-or-teenagers-health (accessed 22 January 2016).

Family Lives (2015) *Underage Drinking*. London: Family Lives. Available at: http://www.familylives.org.uk/advice/teenagers/drugs-alcohol/underage-drinking/ (accessed 22 January 2016).

Health and Social Care Information Centre (2013) *Smoking, Drinking and Drug Use among Young People in England – 2012*. Available at: http://www.hscic.gov.uk/searchcatalogue?productid=12096&q=title:#top (accessed 22 January 2016).

Herring R, Bayley M, Hurcombe R (2012) *A Positive Choice: Young People who Drink Little or No Alcohol*. York: Joseph Rowntree Foundation. Available at: https://www.jrf.org.uk/report/positive-choice-young-people-who-drink-little-or-no-alcohol (accessed 22 January 2016).

Institute of Alcohol Studies (2013) *Children, Adolescents and Underage Drinking. Factsheet.* London: IAS. Available at: http://www.ias.org.uk/uploads/pdf/Factsheets/Underage%20drinking%20 factsheet%20December%202013.pdf (accessed 22 January 2016).

Percy A, Wilson J, McCartan C, McCrystal P (2011) *Teenage Drinking Cultures.* York: Joseph Rowntree Foundation. Available at: https://www.jrf.org.uk/report/teenage-drinking-cultures (accessed 22 January 2016).

Royal College of Paediatrics and Child Health (2015) *Personal Child Health Record.* London: RCPCH. Available at: http://www.rcpch.ac.uk/improving-child-health/public-health/personal-child-health-record/personal-child-health-record (accessed 22 January 2016).

Scottish Government (2015) *Licensing (Scotland) Act 2005 – Section 142: Guidance for Licensing Boards and Local Authorities.* Edinburgh: Scottish Government. Available at: http://www.gov. scot/Publications/2007/04/13093458/12 (accessed 22 January 2016).

Tucker J, Miles J, D'Amico E (2013) Cross-lagged associations between substance use-related media exposure and alcohol use during middle school. *Journal of Adolescent Health* 53: 460–464.

World Health Organization (2006) *Youth Violence and Alcohol.* Geneva: WHO. Available at: http:// www.who.int/violence_injury_prevention/violence/world_report/factsheets/fs_youth.pdf (accessed 22 January 2016).

PART 2
Acutely Ill Children

An infant with pyrexia and febrile convulsions resulting from an unknown infection

Tony Long and Amy Lamb

Case outline

Rangi is 9 months old and has been brought to the accident and emergency (A&E) department by ambulance following what appears to have been a febrile convulsion at home. At present he is awake, distressed and hot. His mother is upset and anxious. He has been generally unwell for 36 hours, with a suddenly rising temperature and a cough. His mother had taken him to the general practice surgery where a viral illness had been diagnosed, and she had been advised to give him plenty of fluids and to give him paracetamol when needed. An hour ago, when clearly pyrexial, he had lost consciousness, his body became stiff, and his arms and legs began to twitch. His eyes rolled back showing the whites. His mother, believing that he was about to die, had called an ambulance. Within minutes, Rangi relaxed, regained consciousness, and although still drowsy became upset. This was the first time that a convulsion had been observed by Rangi's mother.

1 Stop for a moment and think about the scenario that is presented to staff in the department as the paramedics bring Rangi into the department.

A You probably tried to imagine a distraught parent and an uncooperative child, the only witness to what happened being the mother who is frightened and unsure about what is going on. The professionals in the department will be looking and listening for clues immediately to help them to make a diagnosis and to discern if any immediate threats are present.

2 What is a febrile convulsion?

A A febrile convulsion is a generalized seizure in young children occurring in conjunction with a high temperature that is not caused by a central nervous system infection. The case described here is a fairly classical presentation of a febrile convulsion. Although the peak incidence is between 18 and 24 months, they can occur at any time between

6 months and 5 years (American Academy of Pediatrics Subcommittee on Febrile Seizures 2011). Febrile convulsions may be seen in about 2.5–5 per cent of children in the UK (NHS Choices 2014) or in Ireland (Health Service Executive 2014). The mechanism is not clear, but a family history of febrile convulsions approximately doubles the risk of occurrence.

3   See the typology of febrile convulsions (or seizures, or fits – the terminology is often used interchangeably, Figure 4.1). How would you categorize this case, at least initially?

A   This seems to be the first occurrence, and although Rangi's temperature was not taken at the time, from his mother's report it is clear that he was more than usually pyrexial. Generally seizures associated with fever, in a child who has previously had seizures without being pyrexial, are not described as febrile convulsions, but as *convulsions with fever*. Seizures during fever in those who have central nervous system abnormalities are not usually considered to be simple febrile seizures.

4   What do you think are the main issues to be considered in the assessment of Rangi's condition on reception into the department?

A   The medical diagnosis of febrile convulsion is based upon clinical history and observation. Physical examination cannot confirm the diagnosis, but it will often detect signs of the underlying cause of the fever – usually an infection, but occasionally other problems such as neurofibromatosis. It is important to exclude intracranial infection (meningitis or encephalitis), although these are becoming more rare since vaccination has been introduced (National Institute of Health and Care Excellence [NICE] 2007, 2013a). It is important, then, to be thorough and systematic in assessment. The Royal College of Nursing (RCN 2013) states that 100 infants each year in the UK die from infection, and that improved recognition, evaluation and treatment of febrile illness could make a significant improvement on this.

Febrile convulsions

Simple febrile convulsions

Generalized tonic-clonic seizures lasting less than 15 minutes that do not recur within the same febrile illness.

Complex febrile convulsions

Any of the following are diagnostic

- Focal features at onset or during the seizure
- Duration of more than 15 minutes
- Recurrence within the same febrile illness
- Incomplete recovery within 1 hour

Febrile status epilepticus

Febrile convulsion lasting more than 30 minutes

Figure 4.1 Typology of febrile convulsions

CLINICAL ASSESSMENT

Temperature, heart rate, respiratory rate, and capillary refill time have all been shown to be vital criteria for effective clinical decision-making for children with febrile illness (NICE 2007, 2013a). An assessment will be made using the AIMS ABCDE system (Greater Manchester Critical Care Institute 2013).

- **A** (Airway). The airway is clear but the throat is red and inflamed.
- **B** (Breathing). The respiratory rate is raised, but Rangi is hot and upset. Auscultation of the chest is difficult under such circumstances, but the lungs seem to be clear.
- **C** (Circulation). Rangi has a raised heart rate, but, again, this is consistent with his high temperature and distress. Capillary refill is normal. The blood pressure is difficult to measure but the nurses and Rangi's mother manage to calm him sufficiently for a credible reading, which is within acceptable limits.
- **D** (Disability). Rangi has regained consciousness with no deficit.
- **E** (Exposure). Rangi has been stripped to minimal clothing to allow him to cool, and examination of the throat and ears shows evidence of infection, with a red, inflamed throat and bulging right eardrum. Otherwise, he appears to be healthy. A urine sample is tested for leucocytes, nitrates and protein, but the test proves negative.

Health professionals must listen to parental explanation of the history of the problem and their concerns about the severity of their child's illness. Parents recognize changes and abnormalities in their child's demeanour and behaviour better than any doctor or nurse. A wise motto is offered by the Greater Manchester Critical Care Skills Institute (2013): ignore parental concerns at your peril. The discovery of the ear and throat problem correlates with parental reports of a cough and Rangi pulling at his ear. A diagnosis of viral throat and ear infection (otitis media) is made.

5 **Now that the assessment has shown no immediate danger to life and no other injury or illness to that already suspected, what would you do about the three main problems: pyrexia, the cause of the pyrexia and the mother's information needs in case of further episodes? Try to list what you would do for each of these.**

(A) ## PYREXIA

The physiology of temperature regulation

The physiology of maintaining homeostasis is complex, involving several body systems and feedback mechanisms, and regulation of temperature is part of this. The hypothalamus, a small area of grey matter deep in the brain in the floor of the third ventricle, plays a central role in regulating core body temperature (as well as fluid balance, sleep, appetite and emotions). Changes in temperature are sensed both by peripheral temperature sensors from the skin and the visceral organs and by thermoreceptors in the hypothalamus itself (Figure 4.2). The hypothalamus is able to cause the body to

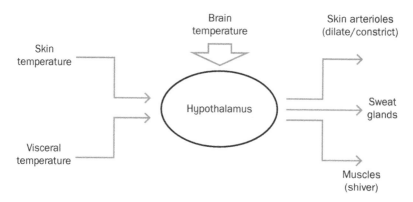

Figure 4.2 The physiology of fever

produce and conserve heat through peripheral vasoconstriction and shivering, or to lose heat by sweating and peripheral vasodilation.

Pyrogens such as bacterial endotoxins and viruses can cause the physiological temperature setting in the hypothalamus to reset to a higher level, preventing action to reduce core temperature until a higher temperature is experienced. Since the hypothalamus is caused by pyrogens to recognize this warmer blood as being below the required temperature set for the body it activates mechanisms to increase the core temperature further. This results in fever (Casey 2000; RCN 2013). Since infants have immature temperature regulatory ability (particularly, having imperfect sensory ability and being unable to sweat or to shiver) they are at particular risk of excesses of heat or cold.

6   **What is the evidence about detection of fever?**

A   The evidence suggests that for children from 1 month to 5 years body temperature should be measured either by electronic thermometer in the axilla, or by infra-red tympanic thermometer (NICE 2013a). In Rangi's case, tympanic membrane temperature can be recorded in his left ear (only). Parental reports of their child developing a fever should be taken seriously (NICE 2007), so the nurse would record the temperature again. Oral and rectal temperature recording should not be made in children up to 5 years, and forehead chemical thermometers should not be used since they are not reliable (NICE 2007).

7   **What antipyretic medication would you expect to give?**

A   Antipyretics such as paracetamol and ibuprofen do not act to prevent convulsions (World Health Organization 2014). However, they should still be given for the patient's comfort since pyrexia is clearly unpleasant and distressing. Either paracetamol or ibuprofen may be given (though not simultaneously) for as long as the child remains distressed (RCN 2013). If one seems not to work, then it is worth trying the other (alone) first before moving on to alternate drugs to cover for recurrence of distress before the next dose of the main medicine (NICE 2013a).

8 What intervention is needed for the ear and throat infection?

A This is thought to be a case of a viral infection, so no other medical treatment is required. However, if it had been considered to be a bacterial infection, then a course of antibiotics would have been prescribed. Specific infections may require particular antimicrobial regimes.

Information for the family

Since a clear focus was found for the underlying infection, Rangi will probably be sent home after a brief period of observation and treatment: perhaps once 6 to 12 hours have gone by after the last convulsion. This practice differs from hospital to hospital. His family will need clear information and instructions for them to feel confident in caring for Rangi.

---

9 Imagine yourself in the place of Rangi's parent. What would worry you? What would you want to know before you went home with him? What questions might you have? Make some notes and see if you can provide the answers.

A **INFORMATION**

No doubt you would want to know why this had happened. A simple explanation of the temperature control mechanism being disturbed by the infection causing the convulsion would help. Clarifying that the terms fit, convulsion and seizure are all used interchangeably in this context might help to resolve confusion.

Perhaps the most frightening aspect of a convulsion for parents is the period of apnoea. Indeed, this is the point at which parents will sometimes shake a child to try to prompt them to breathe. It is important to explain that this is the result of the muscle spasm stiffening the chest briefly, and that no harm occurs. Although the apnoea is brief, it may seem far longer to a distraught parent or carer.

The nurse will also provide information about action to be taken if another convulsion occurs. This will link to a discussion of the likelihood of recurrence. Temperature-taking and learning to understand their own child's limits of pyrexia will be part of the preparation for discharge. Controlling the environmental temperature, recognizing the signs of dehydration, keeping the child hydrated, and checking the child during the night will be advised, and all of this information will be provided in a leaflet as an aide-memoire.

In addition to the safe and effective administration of antipyretics, some families will need to learn how and when to administer rectal or buccal midazolam to terminate longer convulsions. However, these would not normally be used unless a convulsion lasted for more than five minutes.

WORRIES

The first convulsion was terrifying, so you would probably worry first about possible recurrence. Perhaps you would also worry about permanent damage or the possibility

---

Following a first febrile seizure:

- Approximately 30% of children will have one recurrence
- Approximately 15% will have two recurrences
- Approximately 7% will have three or more recurrences
- Approximately 70% of recurrences occur within a year of the first febrile seizure

The risk of recurrence is increased by any of the following:

- A first febrile seizure before the age of 18 months
- Family history of febrile seizures or epilepsy
- Seizure preceded by fever of short duration (less than one hour) or with a temperature of less than 40°C
- A partial seizure
- Multiple seizures during the same febrile episode
- Attendance at a day care nursery

Children who have had a febrile seizure following immunization are no more likely to have a subsequent seizure than children who have had a febrile seizure associated with another cause for fever.

(NICE 2013b)

Figure 4.3 Prevalence and prognosis of febrile seizure

Source: National Institute for Health and Care Excellence 2013b (http://cks.nice.org.uk/febrile-seizure#!backgroundsub:5).

of epilepsy. The nurse would address this by explaining an abbreviated version of the prevalence and prognosis as detailed by NICE (2013b, Figure 4.3). Again, this would be detailed in a booklet.

Key points

- It is always worth making the effort to reflect on what a family's experience of an episode of illness might have been before presenting with a child for professional intervention, since this has an impact on understanding of presenting signs and symptoms.
- Systematic clinical assessment is vital, but it is incomplete without taking into account parental perspectives on the behaviour and demeanour of their child.
- Awareness of, and compliance with, research-informed national guidelines is a crucial part of professional, evidence-based practice.

REFERENCES

American Academy of Pediatrics Subcommittee on Febrile Seizures (2011) Clinical practice guideline – febrile seizures: guideline for the neurodiagnostic evaluation of the child with a simple febrile seizure. *Pediatrics* 127: 389–394 (DOI: 10.1542/peds.2010-3318).

Casey G (2000) Fever management in children. *Nursing Standard* 14(40): 36–40.

Greater Manchester Critical Care Institute (2013) *Paediatric Acute Illness Management (PaedAIM Course Manual).* Available at: http://www.gmccsi.org.uk/aim/paediatric-aim (accessed 22 January 2016).

Health Service Executive (2014) *Febrile Convulsions*. Dublin: HSE. Available at: www.hse.ie/eng/health/az/F/Febrile-seizures/ (accessed 22 January 2016).

National Institute for Health and Care Excellence (2007) *Feverish Illness in Children: Assessment and Initial Management in Children Younger than 5 years*. NICE Clinical Guideline 47. London: NICE. Available at: http://www.nice.org.uk/guidance/cg160/evidence/full-guideline-189990973 (accessed 9 February 2016).

National Institute for Health and Care Excellence (2013a) *Feverish Children – Risk Assessment (Clinical Knowledge Summaries)*. London: NICE. Available at: http://cks.nice.org.uk/feverish-children-risk-assessment#!management (accessed 22 January 2016).

National Institute for Health and Care Excellence (2013b) *Febrile Seizure (Clinical Knowledge Summaries)*. London: NICE. Available at: http://cks.nice.org.uk/febrile-seizure#!background (accessed 16 February 2016).

NHS Choices (2014) *Febrile Seizures*. London: DH. Available at: http://www.nhs.uk/conditions/febrile-convulsions/pages/introduction.aspx (accessed 22 January 2016).

Royal College of Nursing (2013) *Caring for Children with Fever: RCN Good Practice Guidance for Nurses Working with Infants, Children and Young People*. London: RCN. ISBN 978-1-908782-92-2. Available at: https://www2.rcn.org.uk/__data/assets/pdf_file/0008/184895/003267.pdf (accessed 22 January 2016).

World Health Organization (2014) *Management of Febrile Seizures*. Geneva: WHO. Available at: http://www.who.int/mental_health/mhgap/evidence/epilepsy/q3/en/ (accessed 22 January 2016).

CASE STUDY 5
Emergency admission with brittle asthma
Tony Long and Amy Lamb

Case outline

Eight-year-old Asif is admitted by ambulance to the emergency department. He is known to have a severe type of asthma known as brittle asthma. His usual home interventions have had no effect, and he has become gradually worse over the last 24 hours. Asif has been audibly wheezy (heard without a stethoscope) but now his breathing appears to be quiet. It is obvious that Asif is struggling for breath and making use of accessory muscles of respiration. An attached pulse oximeter shows a heart rate of 150 beats per minute and 87 per cent oxygen saturation. The paramedics have applied an oxygen mask and tried to administer nebulized salbutamol, but Asif keeps pulling it down off his face. He is too breathless to speak.

---

1   **Why do asthmatic children have attacks?**

A   An asthmatic attack occurs when environmental triggers stimulate an immune response in the airways. The triggers are commonly dust mite, smoke, perfumes, pollen or ingested particles, although many other substances can exert the effect. An attack can also be triggered by exercise, viral infection or medicines. For example, approximately two-thirds of asthma attacks in school are prompted by rhinovirus infection – the cause of the common cold (European Lung Foundation and European Respiratory Society 2013; European Respiratory Society 2014).

In an asthmatic child, the airways are already hypersensitive to such triggers. The response begins with spasm of the smooth muscle surrounding the bronchi, followed by oedematous inflammation in the lower airways that causes narrowing of the lumen (the hollow in the centre of the tube). Excessive production of mucus then blocks the already narrowed airways. Over time, the airways become scarred and thickened, the immune response is heightened, and the mucus cells become enlarged, producing thicker mucus in greater quantities.

Look in a book of anatomy and physiology to see detailed colour figures of this process, or visit http://www.sign.ac.uk/pdf/SIGN141.pdf (Scottish Intercollegiate Guidelines

Network and British Thoracic Society 2014) or the Asthma Society of Canada website for a clear explanation aimed at parents and patients (http://www.asthma.ca/adults/about/whatIsAsthma.php).

THE IMMEDIATE RESPONSE TO ASIF'S SITUATION

In an emergency situation it is vital to make a rapid assessment and to prioritize problems and actions. The paediatric acute illness management ABCDE approach is often used (Greater Manchester Critical Care Institute 2013).

2   **Make your assessment using the ABCDE approach and then work out what you see as the priorities and what you would do first.**

A Airway – vocalization, airway noises
B Breathing – rate, pattern, depth, chest movement, use of accessory muscles (effort of breathing), oxygen saturation
C Circulation – pallor/cyanosis, pulse rate/rhythm, blood pressure, temperature, urine output, capillary refill rate, skin changes (mottled or cool peripheries)
D Disability – conscious level, interaction with surroundings, pupils, seizures, pain
E Exposure – head-to-toe examination

A   Doing this as an exercise now is one thing, but under the pressure of an emergency, with a possibly moribund child and frantic parents, clear thinking and positive action are essential.

A The airway is clear (the constriction is lower in the respiratory tract).
B Breathing is compromised by the nature of the illness, and urgent action is needed to relieve the obstruction. Oxygen saturation is worryingly low.
C At present the heart rate is raised in response to reduced oxygen content and indicates a struggling patient but an appropriate physiological response. If this were to slow again without improvement in breathing it would signal imminent collapse and possibly death.
D For now, Asif is conscious and able to remove the mask that is psychologically constricting.
E Although the diagnosis seems obvious, a rapid review and history from parents is needed to ensure that there is no additional pathological cause for his condition (for example, anaphylaxis). Thinking ahead, a local anaesthetic gel will be applied in anticipation of venepuncture for blood-testing and likely intravenous infusion or drug administration. Neither of these, however, should delay any immediate necessary interventions.

3   **How serious is Asif's condition?**

A   Asif's condition should be considered life-threatening. This is 'severe asthma' according to the definition offered by the European Respiratory Society and American Thoracic Society (2014). Oxygen saturation (SpO_2) below 92 per cent and heart rate above 125 bpm are signs of severe asthma, but the quiet breathing is especially worrying.

How common is asthma?

Asthma is the most common chronic disease in childhood in the UK and is common throughout the world. In 2014 there were 1.1 million children (1 in 11) in the UK receiving treatment for asthma. (Asthma UK 2014).

Childhood asthma accounted for more than 25,000 episodes of emergency hospital admission in the UK in 2011–2012 (European Respiratory Society 2014).

Asthma prevalence in the UK is high compared to most European countries, and the child mortality rate from asthma has been found to be the worst among eight western European countries (Wolfe et al. 2011).

Figure 5.1 How common is asthma?

This is an indication that air flow is seriously diminished. If there were also a lack of respiratory effort together with drowsiness, this would then also indicate imminent collapse and possibly death. Rapid intervention is essential.

The Scottish Intercollegiate Guidelines Network and British Thoracic Society (2014) will be followed, although regional variations on these are common, particularly regarding drug treatment. See Figure 5.1 for details of the prevalence of asthma.

4   **How will oxygen saturation be improved?**

A   Relieving the obstruction and improving oxygen saturation is the absolute priority. The initial treatment for a child with such a severe attack is to relieve the spasm with bronchodilators, reduce the inflammation with steroid, and provide inhaled oxygen. There is no point in trying to use a salbutamol inhaler since Asif is unable to breathe well enough for this to be inhaled effectively. Repeated doses of nebulized salbutamol together with ipratropium bromide will be given driven by oxygen until the breathing improves. When nebulizers are not being given, oxygen will be provided by a mask since a flow of more than 2L per minute is needed. The effectiveness of each adminis-tration of bronchodilator will be monitored by auscultation and recording the respiratory rate. A dose of oral steroid 1–2 mg/kg will be given if Asif can manage to drink this. If not, then a similar dose will be injected intravenously.

The treatment works, and after two doses of nebulized bronchodilators Asif's oxygen saturation improves to 95 per cent. His heart rate remains high at 128 bpm, and his respiratory rate is 33 breaths per minute, but his breathing is visibly easier. He starts to relax and tolerates an oxygen mask better. On questioning he can make brief replies. There is much less use of accessory mus-cles. The improvement continues and he is transferred to a ward for further management and observation. Asif's treatment is changed from nebulizers to inhalers as his conditions improves in preparation for discharge home.

5   Think now about the nursing care that Asif and his parents will need on the ward until discharged. Identify his likely needs and what you might do to ensure that these are met.

6   How will you ensure his safety?

A   You will, no doubt, have thought to observe Asif and to monitor his vital signs to ensure that his progress continues. Asif has had a rough time of it for nearly two days. He will be tired – even exhausted – from the respiratory effort, hypoxia and lack of sleep. Nurses need to take this physiological need for rest and sleep into account and avoid unnecessary disturbance. The use of electronic monitoring of SpO_2 and heart rate, together with clinical observation skills are helpful in achieving this. However, clinical observation of breathing and auscultation of the chest are essential for ensuring continued recovery even if SpO_2 appears to be satisfactory. Skilful nursing can achieve this without disturbing Asif's rest unduly.

7   What will be done to prevent relapse?

A   The National Institute for Health and Care Excellence (NICE 2013) quality standards provide guidance on the management of asthma throughout these phases. Once he is able to use them effectively, Asif will be encouraged to use his bronchodilator inhaler regularly and to recommence use of his preventer inhaler (for example, beclometasone dipropionate) using a spacer with one puff followed by ten normal breaths. The nurse will check Asif's inhaler technique, since poor technique can be implicated in the development of asthmatic attacks. Once the oxygen saturation is maintained at greater than 92 per cent, Asif will be able to discontinue the oxygen therapy. (A general four-hourly stepdown routine may be followed with ten inhaler puffs per hour for four hours, followed by ten puffs two-hourly for four hours until achieving ten puffs four-hourly.) For a patient to be considered ready to go home, they must be tolerating inhalers at four hourly intervals, the dose of which is required will vary from patient to patient. There is some evidence of the effectiveness of bronchial thermoplasty in reduced exacerbation, reduction in symptoms and improved quality of life in severe asthma (NICE 2011), but this treatment is not yet in common use.

8   Why is psychological care important?

A   Asthma can be frightening no matter how many years it may have been suffered. Being rushed to hospital in an ambulance, experiencing the concern felt by the health professionals and seeing his parents' anxiety and fear may have exerted a psychological impact on Asif. He will want reassurance that he is getting better and that it is safe to go to sleep. Either or both of his parents will be allowed to stay with him, but they, too, will require psychological support. They will realize by now that this could happen again, and they may well have understood the critical point reached by their son before the treatment worked. Asthma typically begins much earlier in life than other chronic diseases, imposing a high lifetime burden on individuals, their carers and the community, and 13% of carers of asthmatic children in Britain reported giving up work to care for their child (European Respiratory Society 2014).

9 **Should you bother about hygiene needs?**

A Although it might not be a priority for Asif, he is likely to have been sweating, coughing, possibly vomiting and not have been able to attend to his hygiene for more than 24 hours. He needs to rest, but a gentle wash – perhaps with the nurse assisting one of his parents – and a change of clothing may make him feel better and also help to draw a line under the critical episode.

10 **What would you do about drinks and food for Asif?**

A Asif is likely to be mildly dehydrated after so much effort, insensible fluid loss and being too breathless to drink, so offering drinks that he likes will help. Despite the time of day, he may be hungry and finally able to consider eating. Since serious asthma is often associated with reactions or allergies to other antigens, it is wise to check again before providing food if Asif has any known food allergies.

INFORMATION NEEDS

Information for Asif and his family will be made available in a leaflet as well as being explained by the nurse. This will include an explanation of the common triggers of worsening asthma (common cold, exercise, changes in the weather, cigarette smoke, allergens such as pollen and pets). It will offer a reminder of the correct use of inhalers, and state clearly when and how to get help either as an emergency or as part of the service offered by the family doctor or asthma nurse.

11 **When can Asif be safely discharged?**

A Using the Scottish Intercollegiate Guidelines Network and British Thoracic Society (2014) guideline, Asif can be discharged when his breathing is stable on 3-4 hourly bronchodilators that he can use at home; when the SpO_2 is better than 94 per cent and when there is primary care support available.

12 **What support will Asif have on discharge?**

A Asif should already have an asthma plan that details the reducing doses of oral steroid and of salbutamol and preventer inhalers. It will indicate expected (normal) peak flow readings.

He will be encouraged to attend appointments with his general practitioner (GP) for regular monitoring of control, growth, and potential side-effects of drugs (especially oral steroids). His GP will maintain an asthma register on which Asif will be entered.

In some areas there may be specialist asthma nurse outreach. Otherwise, a visit from the community children's nurse will have been arranged. This nurse will address any lack of understanding of advice, review Asif's condition and use of inhalers, and discuss potential triggers in the home.

From 1 October 2014, schools must ensure that children have access to a spare emergency inhaler at school (Department of Health 2014). The school nurse will be made aware of Asif's admission to hospital and will take action to ensure that teachers are aware of his needs and how to respond should worsening of the asthma become apparent at school.

A review appointment with a specialist paediatrician will be made for follow-up at about four to six weeks after discharge.

Key points

- Systematic, though sometimes rapid, assessment and prioritizing of a patient's condition is of paramount importance, and this must be repeated to identify improvement or imminent worsening.
- Medical and nursing management takes on board the whole range of a patient's needs; not only those relating to safety. Psychological care is also important.
- A discharge plan must be made that includes referral to other services and briefing of key individuals who will monitor and support ongoing recovery. Important messages will be reinforced through this.

REFERENCES

Asthma UK (2014) *Managing Asthma in Children*. London: Asthma UK. Available at: http://www.asthma.org.uk/advice-children-and-asthma (accessed 22 January 2016).

Department of Health (2014) *Guidance on the Use of Emergency Salbutamol Inhalers in Schools*. London: DH. Available at: https://www.gov.uk/government/publications/emergency-asthma-inhalers-for-use-in-schools (accessed 22 January 2016).

European Lung Foundation and European Respiratory Society (2013) *Lung Health in Europe: Facts and Figures*. Sheffield: ELF. Available at: http://www.europeanlung.org/assets/files/publications/lung_health_in_europe_facts_and_figures_web.pdf (accessed 9 February 2016).

European Respiratory Society (2014) *European Lung White Book*. Sheffield: ERS. Available at: http://www.erswhitebook.org/ (accessed 22 January 2016).

European Respiratory Society and American Thoracic Society (2014) International ERS/ATS guidelines on definition, evaluation and treatment of severe asthma. *European Respiratory Journal* 43: 343–373 (DOI: 10.1183/09031936.00202013). Available at: http://www.thoracic.org/statements/resources/allergy-asthma/Severe-Asthma-CPG-ERJ.pdf (accessed 9 February 2016).

Greater Manchester Critical Care Institute (2013) *Paediatric Acute Illness Management (PaedAIM Course Manual)*. Available at: http://www.gmccsi.org.uk/aim/paediatric-aim (accessed 22 January 2016).

National Institute for Health and Care Excellence (2012) *Bronchial Thermoplasty for Severe Asthma*. London: NICE. Available at: http://www.nice.org.uk/guidance/IPG419 (accessed 22 January 2016).

National Institute for Health and Care Excellence (2011) *Interventional Procedure Overview of Bronchial Thermoplasty for Severe Asthma*. London: NICE. Available at: https://www.nice.org.uk/guidance/ipg419/evidence/overview-438574141 (accessed 9 February 2016).

National Institute for Health and Care Excellence (2013) *Asthma: NICE Quality Standard (QS25)*. London: NICE. Available at: https://www.nice.org.uk/Guidance/QS25 (accessed 9 February 2016).

Scottish Intercollegiate Guidelines Network and British Thoracic Society (2014) *British Guideline on the Management of Asthma. A National Guideline*. Edinburgh: SIGN. Available at: http://www.sign.ac.uk/pdf/SIGN141.pdf (accessed 9 February 2016).

Wolfe I, Cass H, Thompson M, et al. (2011) Improving child health services in the UK: insights from Europe and their implications for the NHS reforms. *British Medical Journal* 342: d1277. Available at: http://dx.doi.org/10.1136/bmj.d1277 (accessed 22 January 2016).

Emergency surgery for appendicitis
Tony Long and Sue Rothwell

Case outline

Sally, aged 14, has suffered from abdominal pain repeatedly for some weeks and has consulted her general practitioner (GP) twice with this problem. On this occasion, she has been brought to the accident and emergency (A&E) department with severe abdominal pain and vomiting, and feeling and looking distinctly unwell. She has arrived with a friend since her parents are at work. She is pale, anxious and clinging to her friend's hand.

---

1   Imagine that you are the triage nurse. What possible causes might you have in mind for abdominal pain in this case? (List these, drawing on your knowledge of anatomy, her gender, her age and other factors.)

A   There are several common causes of abdominal pain in a patient like Sally. The pain might be associated with the menstrual cycle. It might be caused by gastrointestinal infection. Urinary tract infection is another cause, particularly in females because of the shorter urethra and the proximity of the urethral opening to the vagina and the anus. Pregnancy (and especially ectopic pregnancy – a desperately serious situation) should be considered, too, as should pelvic inflammatory disease. Intestinal obstruction would be an immediate threat to life, while worm infestation is possible and of much less urgency. Appendicitis (and consequent peritonitis if the appendix perforates) is, therefore, only one of many possible diagnoses.

2   What action might you want to take immediately to ensure Sally's safety and to start to establish the possible cause?

A   Historically, triage relied on individual nurse's interpretation of a patient's presenting complaint. This could be influenced by a variety of factors, for example the nurse's clinical experience or the nurse's preconceptions. In the early 1990s, a group of practitioners in emergency care devised a system to remove the subjectivity from triage. By utilizing a system of flow charts with specific discriminators even relatively inexperienced nurses are able to prioritize a patient's clinical need.

    The triage nurse would employ the Manchester triage process (Mackway-Jones et al. 2014). Triage is used to determine clinical need. The Manchester triage system consists of a suite of flow charts covering a range of presenting complaints, each consisting of discriminators which, when selected, enable the practitioner to determine the patient's clinical priority. The charts are consistent with one another and, therefore, a number of charts could be utilized for each presentation while still resulting in the same prioritization (Seiger et al. 2014; van Veen et al. 2010). In this case, the practitioner could utilize the abdominal pain in children chart, the diarrhoea and vomiting chart or the unwell child chart. The most important outcome of triage should be that patients who require immediate intervention, especially in life-saving circumstances, should be treated promptly.

Since it is obvious that Sally is conscious, has a clear airway and is not experiencing difficulty in breathing, the next action is to check her circulation. Observations would be made of temperature (in case of infection), pulse, blood pressure, respiration rate and oxygen saturation. The blood sugar level would be established by taking a thumb prick blood sample and using a point-of-care glucose monitoring device. A urine sample would be sought in order that a urine dipstick could be used to check for leucocytes (white blood cells), nitrates and protein in the urine. If positive, this would indicate a urinary tract infection and would require the sample to be sent to the laboratory for urgent microscopy and culture. The urine dipstick would also test for glucose. As with all cases, careful eliciting of the history of the problem is important, giving credence to patients' accounts and to the concerns of parents. A local anaesthetic gel with dressing will be applied in anticipation of the venepuncture.

3 **You need to know if there is any possibility of Sally being pregnant. This can be a sensitive matter, particularly if a teenager is accompanied by a parent. Think about how and when you would tackle this. Identify the benefits and problems of the presence of Sally's friend.**

A Discussion about possible pregnancy and, therefore, of sexual activity in the presence of a parent might be difficult for some teenagers (although not for all) – whether or not there could be cause for concern of pregnancy. You would normally want to ask discreetly but in a straightforward manner that encourages an honest response. The opportunity might be taken while Sally is alone for weighing or to provide a urine specimen. However, severe abdominal pain related to pregnancy could indicate imminent rupture of an ectopic pregnancy, so there is no time to waste, and antibiotics to treat a suspected infection could also have devastating effects on a fetus. A good place to start is to enquire first about the onset of menarche, about regularity of periods, and if one has been missed.

What about Sally's friend? There is evidence that friendship networks are important sources of teenagers' advice, information and decision-making support (Fallon 2010). Sally's friend might know the required information, and might be the means by which Sally would prefer to reveal it. She might be reassured by her friend's presence. On the other hand, the friend might not know, and Sally might prefer to keep it that way. Part of the nurse's skillset is to read the situation, to be responsive to cues and non-verbal messages, to appreciate the probable concerns of the patient, and to be sufficiently confident to broach sensitive topics in an open, direct, yet thoughtful manner (Fallon 2012, Wray & Stewart 2012).

The history, tests and clinical examination indicate that appendicitis is the most likely cause of the abdominal pain. If the patient is not showing signs of the need for immediate surgery, or if the diagnosis remains uncertain, a period of observation for 24 hours is often undertaken to allow, for example, for more certain diagnosis of urinary infection or gynaecological problems to be recognized, or sometimes for the acute episode to subside. The ideal situation is to undertake planned surgery on a patient who is well. In either case, both pharmaceutical and non-pharmaceutical measures will be adopted to control pain.

However, in this case, Sally needs surgery that will be undertaken the following morning. A laparoscopic (minimally invasive or 'keyhole') technique will be used. Her parents are contacted. Her father is able to come to the hospital immediately, and he will also ensure that Sally's friend gets home safely. Sally's mother will visit later.

4 **Make two lists of the care that Sally will need pre-operatively and post-operatively (after return to the ward). Think about both physical and psychological needs.**

A **PRE-OPERATIVE CARE**

As with any patient, it is important that Sally is identified correctly, so, following local policy, she will have an identity bracelet, including personal details and statements of allergies. She and her parents will also require a simple but honest explanation of what is happening to her, the planned surgery, and a rough timetable of events until she goes home.

Sally will have a general anaesthetic, so her stomach needs to be empty before surgery. She will fast for six hours (local practices vary), but will be allowed to drink water until two hours before surgery. This will prevent her becoming dehydrated, but also ensure that water will be absorbed quickly and not pool in the stomach.

There is the possibility of pre-medication being provided to deal with anxiety, but this is not common practice any more. It is, however, standard practice for distraction therapy to be provided. Nurses and play therapists will reduce anxiety and allow for additional modes of communication by engaging in activities appropriate to Sally's age and according to her preferences.

At the required time, Sally will have to don a theatre gown, with hair tied back, nail coverings removed, and non-removable jewellery covered. Consent would need to be obtained either from Sally or one of her parents. A surgical marking form and a pre-operative checklist would need to be completed and checked with the operating theatre staff on transfer to their care.

POST-OPERATIVE CARE

Observation of vital signs will be undertaken frequently at first, reducing in frequency as normal ranges are achieved and remain stable.

Normal, steady respirations and satisfactory oxygen saturation will have been restored before transfer from recovery to the ward. The heart rate and rhythm (together with skin colour) are important as signs of recovery, of bleeding, shock and impending collapse, and of potential infection. Similarly, the temperature will be recorded to watch for additional signs of infection.

As soon as Sally feels able, she will be provided with drinks, both for comfort and to ensure her hydration.

Laparoscopic surgery reduces the handling of intestines and prevents the once-common problem of temporary paralysis of the ileus. This, together with smaller incisions and less pain, means that Sally will be encouraged to eat within hours of the operation. Good nutrition speeds recovery and helps to prevent infection taking hold.

If vomiting is experienced, then intravenous fluids will be administered, and both analgesics and any antibiotics will be delivered by this route.

Sally will probably have two small wounds that will have been closed with subcutaneous sutures (or occasionally staples). Clear dressings are often used so that the wound can be observed without repeated disturbance and possibility of infecting the site.

Although laparoscopic surgery is far less painful than open surgery, pain relief will still be required. Residual carbon dioxide (used to inflate the abdomen to visualize the organs more clearly) can itself be painful. Intravenous morphine will be used initially, but on return to the ward paracetamol or ibuprofen are usually sufficient (sometimes an initial dose of intravenous paracetamol is required). The need for sustained release morphine is exceptional.

As Sally feels able, and with explanation about its importance, she will be encouraged to start to mobilize again, first sitting by the bed, then standing and walking. The abdominal inflammation, the surgery itself and a period of dehydration, lack of appetite and general immobility can all lead to sluggish function of the bowel. Being able to walk to the toilet might be both an incentive to start walking, but also more effective in achieving bowel emptying.

PRE-DISCHARGE PLANNING

Sally will stay in hospital after the operation probably for only 24 hours, although this varies between surgeons and between departments. For some cases that are not straightforward, patients might stay for two days after the day of surgery. Sound pre-discharge planning is essential for a smooth transition to primary care and for swift, complete recovery.

5   **What needs to be included in the plan?**

A   **COMMUNICATION**

A letter will be sent to the GP to inform of the surgery and to ask the GP to continue the care. Different local arrangements may be in place to arrange for a community nursing team to take up the nursing role.

INFORMATION

Printed information will be provided for parents on pain relief, bathing, return to activities, observation of the wound, and return to school. Contact details for advice will be included.

WOUND CARE

The dressings will usually need to be reviewed after about five days. Wounds are often closed with dissolvable sutures that do not require removal, although families require an explanation about this. Unusually, clips or sutures may need to be removed, but the specific need will have been advised in the referral process. If there is local infection, minor dehiscence (opening along the suture line), or other problem, then the community nursing team will be skilled in diagnosing and treating the problem.

TRANSPORT

The nurse will ensure that the family has the means to transport Sally home. If necessary, hospital transport or a taxi might be needed to facilitate this.

RETURN TO SCHOOL

When there is no pain, the wounds have healed and Sally feels up to it, she can return to school. There may be a school nurse who can be made aware of the surgery so as to be ready to check with Sally, to advise teaching staff, and to respond knowledgeably to any problems that arise.

Key points

- Triage is a skilled activity on which identification of the need for urgent treatment is based. It is usually supported by flow charts to guide decision-making.
- Nurses must be prepared to engage in discussion of sensitive topics with children and young people. Ensuring privacy; speaking in direct, honest terms; and being responsive to cues and non-verbal messages are essential aspects of this activity.
- Pre-operative and post-operative care is based on responses to problems and proactive intervention for potential problems. Awareness of the evidence base to support associated clinical decisions is essential.

REFERENCES

Fallon D (2010) Accessing emergency contraception: the role of friends in the adolescent experience. *Sociology of Health & Illness* 32(5): 677–694 (DOI: 10.1111/j.1467-9566.2010.01237.x).

Fallon D (2012) Communicating with young people, in V Lambert, T Long, D Kelleher (eds) *Communication Skills for Children's Nurses*. Maidenhead: Open University Press: pp. 34–48.

Mackway-Jones K, Marsden J, Windle J (eds) (2014) *Emergency Triage: Manchester Triage Group (3rd edn)*. Chichester: John Wiley & Sons.

Seiger N, van Veen M, Almeida H, et al. (2014) Improving the Manchester triage system for pediatric emergency care: an international multicenter study. PLOS One 9(1): e83267 (DOI: 10.1371/journal.pone.0083267).

van Veen M, Teunen-van der Walle VFM, Steyerberg EW, et al. (2010) Repeatability of the Manchester Triage System for children. *Emergency Medicine Journal* 27(7): 512–516 (DOI: 10.1136/emj.2009.077750).

Wray J, Stewart V (2012) Communicating with vulnerable and disadvantaged children, in V Lambert, T Long, D Kelleher (eds) *Communication Skills for Children's Nurses*. Maidenhead: Open University Press: pp. 105–118.

PART 3
Critically Ill Children

Respiratory distress syndrome (RDS) in a neonate

Michaela Barnard and Louise Weaver-Lowe

Case outline

Jamie was born at 29 weeks' gestation weighing 1.3 kg. He required resuscitation and intubation at birth. He had two doses of surfactant and continued on ventilation for three weeks. Jamie is now 6 weeks old. He is having nasal CPAP (continuous positive airway pressure) with variable oxygen requirements of 25–35 per cent. He has been slowly increasing his enteral feeds by orogastric tube and is gradually gaining weight; he recently weighed 2.1 kg. During routine nursing care, Jamie is noted to have increased work of breathing, a respiratory rate of 66 breaths per minute but with some notable periods of apnoea. He has respiratory distress syndrome (RDS).

---

1 **What signs of increased work of breathing would you look for in a neonate?**

A The first indicator of increased work of breathing is tachypnoea. It is crucial to have an understanding of normal limits for physiological observations in a neonate according to their corrected gestation. Jamie is now at a corrected gestation of 35 weeks, so he is expected to have a respiratory rate of 40–60 breaths per minute. Jamie should then have a respiratory assessment to identify any further signs of increased work of breathing. Common signs in a neonate include intercostal, lower costal or sternal recession; nasal flaring; tracheal tug; cyanosis and an expiratory grunt. An expiratory grunt is respiratory noise observed primarily in neonates with RDS. It is a coping mechanism to prevent alveolar collapse, as the baby expires against a closed glottis (Meeks et al. 2010).

2 **Think about what should be done upon finding this change in Jamie's clinical condition.**

A Jamie's deteriorating condition and respiratory distress would need to be reported to either an advanced neonatal nurse practitioner (ANNP) or a doctor. Jamie would need to be closely observed. As he is already a high-dependency baby requiring CPAP, he would require continuous monitoring of heart rate, respiratory rate, oxygen saturation, blood pressure and temperature. Jamie would need to be observed for sustained or further deteriorating work of breathing. See Figure 7.1 for common causes of RDS in neonates.

Common causes of RDS in neonates

- Surfactant deficient lung disease
- Pneumothorax
- Aspiration
- Chronic lung disease
- Anaemia
- Infection

Figure 7.1 Common causes of respiratory distress syndrome (RDS)

CPAP: CONTINUOUS POSITIVE AIRWAY PRESSURE

The two main indications for CPAP are following extubation and mild to moderate respiratory distress. The purpose of CPAP is to prevent complete collapse of the alveoli, similar to the expiratory grunt that neonates will naturally adopt in respiratory distress. When CPAP is used in mild to moderate RDS, signs of work of breathing and respiratory rate should decrease. Continuous positive airway pressure is delivered through less invasive equipment than full ventilation, requiring either soft prongs or a mask to maintain a seal around the nose (Figure 7.2). The prongs or mask are kept in place by

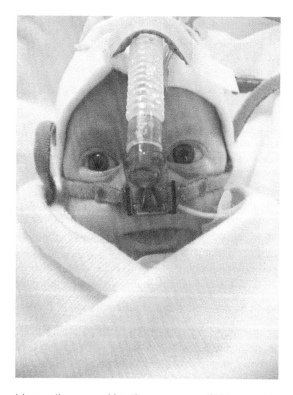

Figure 7.2 Infant receiving continuous positive airway pressure (CPAP) treatment

strapping to a purpose-made hat. The soft prongs used to obtain a seal around the nares can cause pressure to the delicate skin and mucosa. Careful observation of the skin and regular relief of pressure is required to ensure skin integrity is maintained.

3   **What is apnoea of prematurity?**

A   Apnoea can be defined as cessation of breathing for 6 seconds or more (Levene et al. 2008). Apnoea of prematurity is a result of immature respiratory control systems in the midbrain and brainstem. It is an extremely common condition in neonates of less than 34 weeks' gestation. In neonates that are less than 26 weeks' gestation, it is almost an expected event. As a baby born at 29 weeks' gestation, Jamie is likely to have a history of apnoea. This condition normally resolves when infants reach 32–34 weeks' gestation but may persist in infants that develop chronic lung disease (CLD). Apnoea can occur in more mature infants and examination is required to investigate possible causes, such as sepsis, upper airway obstruction, anaemia, hypoglycaemia and current respiratory illness such as pneumonia.

A prophylactic approach is taken to manage apnoea of prematurity. Babies of less than 32 weeks' gestation who are not ventilated, are on CPAP, or are weaning from the ventilator should be commenced on prophylaxis. Caffeine citrate is often the medication of choice, although other methylxanthines such as aminophylline or theophylline can be used. Caffeine acts as a respiratory stimulant, increasing minute volume and reducing diaphragmatic fatigue.

An initial loading dose of 20 mg/kg of caffeine citrate is required. This should be followed by a maintenance dose of 5–10 mg/kg of caffeine citrate once every 24 hours. Caffeine citrate can be administered either by slow intravenous injection or orally: the dosage is the same by either route.

Calculation exercise

Calculate the correct loading and maintenance doses of caffeine citrate for Jamie. Decide whether he should be prescribed an oral or intravenous dose in the present circumstances.

The answer is given at the end of this case on p. 55.

Jamie is reviewed by an ANNP. A clinical assessment is undertaken including auscultation of the chest. Capillary blood gas is checked, and a chest x-ray is ordered (CXR). The capillary blood gas shows that Jamie has a respiratory acidosis, with a low pH and raised pCO_2. This indicates that his increased work of breathing has been unsuccessful in increasing expiration of carbon dioxide.

When a baby has RDS, the chest x-ray is likely to show under-inflation of the lungs and a visible pattern over the lungs often referred to as a 'ground glass' appearance.

Positioning of the nasogastric or orogastric tube is normally confirmed during review of CXR as displacement of enteral feeding tubes can cause respiratory problems.

Respiratory distress syndrome of the newborn is an acute lung disease most often caused by surfactant deficiency, which leads to alveolar collapse. Refer to Part 5, Case 14 for more information on surfactant deficiency.

4   **What nursing care is needed now for Jamie using a prioritized approach?**

A   The primary concern when caring for Jamie is observation and management of his airway and breathing. Poor positioning of a baby can affect the patency of the airway. Babies have poor muscle tone in the face, neck and mouth, and if Jamie's neck is over-extended or his head is in a chin-on-chest position, his tongue may block or partially block the airway. Jamie's head should be in a neutral position allowing for maximum lung expansion. He will be monitored continuously and close observation of respiratory rate, oxygen saturation and work of breathing must continue. It may be necessary to increase the amount of supplemental oxygen slightly following Jamie's deterioration. Any further deterioration will need to be reported to the ANNP or doctor.

Nursing care for Jamie's other needs should continue. The ANNP may decide in view of the acute respiratory deterioration that enteral feeding should cease initially while Jamie's breathing is stabilized. Jamie will already have intravenous access, therefore intravenous fluids can be commenced. Jamie should be subjected to minimal handling, and caring tasks should be clustered. This will help to prevent undue disturbance causing fluctuations in heart rate, respiratory rate and oxygen saturation (Zeiner et al. 2015).

Jamie's parents should be informed about his deterioration in condition and what the plan of treatment and care will be. This will be an anxious time for them as Jamie has made gradual improvements in his ability to breath with less invasive interventions. They will be concerned that Jamie may deteriorate further, needing re-intubation, and they are likely to have ongoing concerns about the long-term impact of continuing respiratory problems.

Two hours later, Jamie's monitor is alarming and it is observed that his oxygen saturation is falling steadily; currently at 82 per cent. He is pale and becoming cyanosed around the lips. His heart rate is 87 bpm and falling. Jamie quickly becomes apnoeic and progresses into respiratory arrest with a heart rate of 55 bpm.

---

5   **This is a situation requiring urgent action. As the student nurse at the side of the incubator, what should you do? What would you expect other health professionals to do?**

A   Babies deteriorate very quickly and can progress from respiratory distress to respiratory arrest in minutes with little warning. Close observation, and quick assessment and action are required. Naturally, the nurse should call for help immediately. The resuscitation trolley with emergency medications should be brought to the bed space. Cardiac arrest teams are not normally called to the neonatal intensive care unit (NICU) due to the sufficient amount of skilled medical and nursing staff able to deal with any neonatal emergency. Newborn life support (NLS) should be commenced using the algorithm from the UK Resuscitation Council (2015). Newborn life support comprises the following elements:

- drying and covering the newborn baby to conserve heat
- assessing the need for any intervention
- opening the airway
- aerating the lung
- rescue breathing
- chest compression
- administration of drugs (rarely).

Jamie is not a newborn who needs to be dried. Jamie should be repositioned in the incubator to allow for maximal access to his airway. The algorithm should start at assessment of breathing and heart rate. The airway should be in the neutral position. If Jamie is gasping or not breathing, five inflation breaths should be given using the mask and Neopuff. Rapid reassessment should be made before consideration of Jamie's bradycardia. If there is no increase in heart rate and it remains below 60 bpm, then chest compressions should be commenced, with three compressions to each breath. Emergency drugs are used only in rare circumstances and in the instance that there is no significant cardiac output despite resuscitative efforts. Emergency drugs that may be used include adrenaline (1:10,000 solution), sodium bicarbonate and 10 per cent dextrose. Such emergency events in neonatal care are normally respiratory in nature unless there is an underlying cardiac abnormality. Babies will normally respond quickly and successfully to cardiopulmonary resuscitation (CPR) on the NICU. Unlike adults, need for cardiac compressions in neonates does not necessarily signify a grave situation.

NEOPUFF

The Neopuff and attached mask is a piece of equipment unique to neonatal care (Figure 7.3). It delivers a breath at a predetermined oxygen/air concentration and pressure by the user obscuring a hole at the head of the mask/tubing with their thumb. This reduces the incidence of hyperoxia and barotrauma in the preterm infant.

The nurse's role in a CPR situation such as Jamie's may be to deliver respiratory support or chest compressions. Documentation of resuscitation needs to be undertaken contemporaneously as many interventions, treatment decisions and medications may be given in a short time period (Nursing and Midwifery Council 2015). A multidisciplinary approach is needed in a CPR situation, with clear leadership guiding each member's roles.

Jamie's parents may have been witness to his deterioration and collapse. If parents are not on the NICU, they should be contacted urgently to attend the unit. The decision regarding whether parents stay during resuscitation has been debated, and in some instances it may be agreed that parents can stay (Sawyer et al. 2015). Whether parents stay and witness the resuscitation or wait in a family room, they should be accom-

(a)

(b)

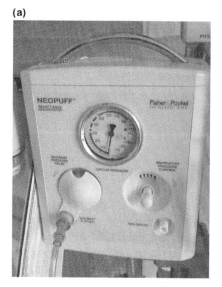
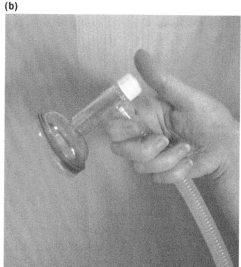

Figure 7.3 (a) Neopuff machine and (b) mask

panied by a nurse and supported. Parents who witness resuscitation may experience negative emotions and some level of trauma. Explanation during the procedure and debriefing afterwards may reduce the incidence of these complications. Curtains or screens should be used to protect Jamie's privacy and dignity. Care and support should also be provided for other parents visiting their babies in the unit who see that an emergency is occurring.

> Jamie was intubated during resuscitation and is now receiving positive pressure ventilation. The treatment plan is to observe his spontaneous respiratory effort, blood gases and any episodes of bradycardia and desaturation. If Jamie remains stable he will be extubated back onto nasal CPAP.

6 **Now that Jamie is stabilized following intubation, what are the care considerations after the resuscitation?**

A To facilitate good outcomes for any baby with RDS, supportive care should be provided including maintenance of a thermo-neutral environment, good nutritional support, appropriate fluid management, management of ductus arteriosus and maintenance of tissue perfusion through circulatory support (Sweet et al. 2013). Jamie will be moved from the high-dependency area to the intensive care area. Jamie should be re-positioned comfortably in the incubator with all incubator doors secure. It is likely that the exposure required during CPR will have resulted in Jamie's core temperature having reduced. Hypothermia in itself can cause respiratory distress, so it is vital to warm Jamie as soon as possible to maintain respiratory stability. Temperature readings should be taken immediately and strategies for warming put into place, such as increased incubator temperature, humidity and a warming mattress. Continuous skin temperature monitoring can be commenced.

A CXR should be taken to check positioning of Jamie's endotracheal tube (ETT). The nurse should auscultate his lungs to obtain a new baseline for air entry and respiratory sounds bilaterally. This will facilitate future assessments of improvement or deterioration in air entry. Continuous monitoring of Jamie's physiological observations should be maintained.

When Jamie is stable, explanations of resuscitation, planned care and new equipment should be discussed in partnership with his parents. His parents will be anxious about the events that have occurred, the likelihood of repetition, and what this means regarding his recovery. Honest and open communication should be central to any discussions with opportunity for dialogue and questions from the family. Parents should be encouraged to touch and talk to Jamie, which should reduce both baby and parental stress levels.

Answer to calculation exercise

The caffeine loading dose should be 42 mg. The maintenance dose should be between 10.5–21 mg once daily. The most appropriate route for Jamie would be intravenous.

Key points

- The specific physiology of neonates demands amended approaches to assessment and treatment, and respiratory issues predominate.
- Prematurity brings additional problems requiring supportive management until the baby develops further. Some of these are partially predictable, so prophylactic intervention is taken.
- The drugs used to treat sick neonates may not be familiar to non-specialists, and doses tend to be much smaller than usual, requiring particularly accurate calculation: an issue that applies to management of fluid requirements, too.

REFERENCES

Levene MI, Tudehope DI, Sinha S (2008) *Essential Neonatal Medicine (4th edn)*. Malden, MA: Blackwell Publishing.

Meeks M, Hallsworth M, Yeo H (2010) *Nursing the Neonate (2nd edn)*. Chichester: Wiley-Blackwell.

Nursing and Midwifery Council (2015) *The Code. Professional Standards of Practice and Behaviour for Nurses and Midwives*. London: NMC. Available at: http://www.nmc.org.uk/globalassets/sitedocuments/nmc-publications/revised-new-nmc-code.pdf (accessed 23 January 2016).

Resuscitation Council (UK) (2015) *Newborn Life Support*. London: Resuscitation Council. Available at: https://www.resus.org.uk/resuscitation-guidelines/resuscitation-and-support-of-transition-of-babies-at-birth/ (accessed 23 January 2016).

Sawyer A, Ayers S, Bertullies S, et al. (2015) Providing immediate neonatal care and resuscitation at birth beside the mother: parents' views, a qualitative study. *British Medical Journal Open* 5: e008495 (DOI:10.1136/bmjopen-2015-008495).

Sweet D G, Carnielli V, Greisen G, et al. (2013) European consensus guidelines on the management of neonatal respiratory distress syndrome in preterm infants – 2013 update. *Neonatology* 103: 353–368.

Zeiner V, Storm H, Doheney KK (2015) Preterm infants' behaviors and skin conductance responses to nurse handling in the NICU. *Journal of Maternal-Fetal and Neonatal Medicine* October 6: 1–6 (Epub ahead of print) (DOI: 10.3109/14767058.2015.1092959).

A 2-year-old toddler who has sustained a head injury
Tony Long and Amy Lamb

Case outline

Two-year-old Jess was playing out unsupervised by an adult when she was hit by a car driven at 20 mph. The distraught driver stopped, called an ambulance and offered what little first aid could be remembered under the circumstances. Jess is brought to the emergency department by paramedics who had been able to establish from witnesses and their own observations that she had been standing when hit by the car, so taking the full force of the impact on her head, and landed on a hard tarmac surface. It was unclear if she had lost consciousness, but she had not vomited. There was a large, bleeding bump on her forehead, and grazes on her face and arms. She is three-point immobilized with a collar to stabilize the cervical spine, blocks on either side of the head to prevent further movement, and tape across the forehead and chin.

---

1 **A vital aspect of ensuring positive outcomes in trauma care is an effective handover from paramedics to emergency department staff. What information would the receiving trauma team seek from the paramedics?**

A An agreed handover template structures the interaction and can reduce information loss (Evans et al. 2010). A version of the MIST structured report would be used (Figure 8.1); MIST stands for Mechanism of the injury; Injuries sustained (or Injury pattern); Signs and symptoms (observations); and Treatment (applied so far). Sometime this is prefixed by AT (Age and Time of incident) – 'AT MIST'. The paramedic report would be short and factual – no more than 30 seconds, and the whole trauma team would listen.

All of this helps the team to understand what has happened and points towards likely diagnoses and immediate treatment needs. Two additional elements are included in the report that are of great importance in this case: assessment of the level of consciousness and a brief test following the acronym 'AVPU' that rates the responsiveness of a patient.

AVPU

- Alert – the patient is alert and responsive without stimulus.
- Voice – the patient responds to spoken commands ('Squeeze my hands').

MIST handover

Mechanism of injury

Hit by a car at low speed. Witnesses reported that she was standing up and took the impact on her head. Fell onto tarmac.

Injuries sustained

Blunt trauma. Obvious head injury with bleeding and bulge. No other obvious fractures. Otherwise minor grazes.

Signs and symptoms

Pulse: 125. Respirations: 30 (distressed). SpO_2: 96% with oxygen mask. Glasgow Coma Scale score: 10. Responsive to voice.

Treatment

Three-point immobilization of neck. Unable to site intravenous cannula.

Figure 8.1 MIST (Mechanism of the injury; Injuries sustained [or Injury pattern]; Signs and symptoms [observations]; and Treatment [applied so far]) handover

- Pain – although not responsive to voice, the patient responds to pain (for example: groaning when a fracture site is disturbed).
- Unresponsive – no response can be elicited at all.

GLASGOW COMA SCALE (GCS)

Although AVPU is a helpful rapid assessment a more precise and reliable measure is the GCS. Although important measures of vital signs and pupillary responses add helpful diagnostic data, the main element of the scale tests eye, verbal and motor responses. The individual and collective scores of these are recorded. The highest score is 15 (fully awake with no deficit), whereas the lowest possible score is 3 (indicating either death or deep coma, Table 8.1). Threshold scores prompt various interventions for differing groups of patients.

Application of the GCS to young children is problematic – especially if language skills are insufficient – so a modified version is often used: the Paediatric GCS (PGCS, Table 8.2).

Decerebrate and decorticate responses

The decorticate response is characterized by clenched fists, with fingers, wrists and elbows stiffly flexed, and the arms flexed across the chest. The legs are extended and

Table 8.1 Degrees of injury according to the Glasgow Coma Scale

15	*≥13*	*9–12*	*≤8*	*3*
(Normal)	Mild	Moderate	Severe	(Deep coma)

Adapted from: Scottish Intercollegiate Guidelines Network (SIGN) 2009.

Table 8.2 Comparison of Glasgow Coma Scale (GCS) and Paediatric Glasgow Coma Scale (PGCS)

		1	2	3	4	5	6
Eye	GCS	Does not open eyes	Opens eyes in response to painful stimuli	Opens eyes in response to voice – for child 'to speech'	Opens eyes spontaneously		
	PGCS						
Verbal	GCS	No verbal response	Incomprehensible sounds	Utters inappropriate words	Confused, disorientated	Oriented, converses normally	
	PGCS	Makes no sounds	Inconsolable agitated	Inconsistently inconsolable moaning	Cries but inconsolable, inappropriate interactions	Smiles, orients to sounds, follows objects, interacts	
Motor	GCS	Makes no movement	Extension to painful stimuli (decerebrate response)	Abnormal flexion to painful stimuli (decorticate response)	Flexion/ withdrawal to painful stimuli	Localizes painful stimuli	Obeys commands
	PGCS	No motor response	Extension to pain (decerebrate response)	Abnormal flexion to pain for an infant (decorticate response)	Infant withdraws from pain	Infant withdraws from touch	Infant moves spontaneously or purposefully

the body is generally rigid. This is a sign of damage or pressure in the cerebral hemi-spheres and possibly the midbrain.

The decerebrate response is typified by the arms and legs being extended out, with neck arched back and the toes pointed downwards. The same rigidity is found.

Activity

Look up the terms 'decerebrate' and 'decorticate' online to find a diagram or picture of each, and check against the descriptions above.

Although both of these responses indicate brain injury, the decerebrate response is more concerning, often indicating damage to the brain stem. However, decorticate responses can deteriorate into decerebrate responses as intracranial pressure increases. Both show the possibility of pressure squeezing the brain across structures in the skull, damaging brain tissues and, in the case of tonsillar herniation (or 'coning') compressing the brain stem with potentially fatal consequences.

At 2 years of age, Jess is on the cusp of these movements being considered relevant since in younger children such responses are not necessarily seen. An overall assessment of Jess is that she has a moderate brain injury, is needing oxygen to keep a satisfactory SpO_2, has tachycardia and a raised respiratory rate (possibly from pain and distress).

Following the handover from the paramedics, the emergency department staff undertake a more detailed ABCDE assessment (Greater Manchester Critical Care Institute 2013).

A (Airway) The airway is clear and already protected.
B (Breathing) The respiratory rate is elevated, and oxygen is needed to maintain saturation. No chest injuries found on examination (flail chest or pneumothorax, for example).
C (Circulation) There is tachycardia. Capillary refill is a little slow. It is difficult to record the blood pressure since Jess is so agitated.
D (Disability) The PGCS is repeated. The score is still 10. The right pupil is slightly sluggish in response to light, although the pupils are of equal size.
E (Exposure) Full examination shows no other significant injuries. Although Jess is experiencing pain, no morphine will be given since assessment of her state is already difficult.

IMMEDIATE MANAGEMENT

The trauma team is called immediately. Typically, this might include the emergency department consultant if not already in attendance, two trauma nurses, the medical registrar for surgery, the registrar for anaesthetics, the radiographer and the radiologist. This list is not exhaustive and may differ from hospital to hospital (The neurosurgeon might be called, but often this is delayed until the computed tomography [CT] result is known).

2 **Stop and think for a moment about why each of these people might be called and what their role might be in Jess's treatment and care. Consider carefully what the nursing contribution will be.**

A The emergency department consultant and nurses specialize in assessing and treating children with trauma with the associated complexity of the situation, often with insufficient information, and needing to make rapid evaluation and re-assessment of priorities. A surgeon is present to assess immediate life-threatening surgical emergencies, and the anaesthetist is essential for the immediate airway management (remember that the three-point immobilization complicates this). Guidelines from the National Institute for Health and Care Excellence (NICE 2014: 9) list a number of criteria that should lead to a child with a head injury having a CT head scan undertaken within 1 hour of the injury being sustained. Jess meets one of these: 'on initial emergency department assessment, GCS less than 14, or for children under 1 year GCS (paediatric) less than 15'. Accordingly, the radiologist who will undertake the scan and the radiologist who will interpret the result need to be available.

Two intravenous cannulae would be sited in anticipation of the need for blood samples and for the administration of fluids and drugs. The nurses will use their skills to achieve this – with an uncooperative child and possibly rapidly evolving demands for other interventions. Intravenous fluid will be delivered in small aliquots to ensure that any clots that have formed are not dislodged and to ensure that clotting agents in the blood are not diluted. Arrangements for safe transfer to the scanner have to be made. If parents or other family members have accompanied the patient, then they also need attention, with information appropriate to a non-professional, explanations of what is happening and what else might happen, and reassurance to the extent that this is appropriate. The nurse might also elicit further information about the circumstances of the accident, but with caution since this could be a potential safeguarding issue.

The CT scan reveals that there is no penetrating injury, with uncertainty as to a fracture, but with a definite, small extradural haematoma. Repeated neurological observations, however, show dilation of the right pupil: a sign of increasing intracranial pressure. Mannitol is infused to draw fluid from the brain and reduce the pressure. The neurosurgeon is consulted, judges that surgery is not required, and recommends conservative treatment. Jess is transferred to the intensive care unit.

Jess is sedated, intubated, and ventilated for 24 hours. Drugs are administered to paralyse her muscles so that she does not make respiratory efforts against the ventilator. This sedation and ventilation allows for increased cerebral oxygenation and control of cerebral blood pressure. Controlling a normal arterial concentration of carbon dioxide (normocapnia) helps to normalize intracranial pressure since too high a concentration dilates cerebral blood vessels and increases pressure.

Hydration is provided by intravenous means, but a careful record is kept of fluid balance. Mannitol is an osmotic diuretic and is often used in patients with head injuries to treat cerebral oedema. All of this is aimed at reducing intracranial pressure while the effects of the injury subside. This care will be provided in the paediatric intensive care unit. Critical care units are the best place to find expert fundamental nursing care as well as the more intense and sometimes technical aspects of nursing.

While Jess is immobile it is vital to care for her skin. Pressure sores can develop just as in adults, so regular movement and use of pressure-relieving aids are employed. Modern beds in intensive care units have inbuilt pressure-relieving systems. Mouth care is needed, as is general hygienic care. Despite Jess being sedated and paralysed, the nurses will talk to her and explain before doing anything to her. Her immediate family will be allowed and encouraged to visit and to talk to her. Reading stories to her may be easier for some visitors. Observations of oxygen saturation, blood pressure and heart rate will be maintained, although neurological observation will be limited by the sedation and paralysis.

Once the intracranial pressure has been controlled and ventilatory support is no longer needed, and following discussion with the multidisciplinary team (particularly neurosurgeons and intensivists), the sedation and paralysing agent will be progressively reduced so that Jess will be allowed to regain consciousness and movement. This will enable complete neurological assessment, as well as facilitating review of any further injuries as a result of the accident. Patients such as Jess often recover well, require minimal outpatient services, and return to normal activities in a short space of time.

SAFEGUARDING

3   **Why would this case be a matter for safeguarding processes to be followed?**

A   The circumstances of Jess's accident are concerning. A 2 year old should not be playing out unsupervised, especially near a road. It is estimated that 25–30 per cent of children aged under 2 years who are hospitalized with head injury have an abusive head injury (NICE 2014: 4). In this case, the head injury was not caused deliberately, but it is possible that neglectful parenting contributed to the event. This requires careful and sensitive investigation.

4   **What guidelines and support are available for staff in such circumstances?**

A   All NHS staff receive regular training and updating in safeguarding, as do nursing students. This training includes knowing what to report and to whom, and the potential sources of support and advice. The hospital that has received Jess will have a named nurse for safeguarding children and a named doctor for safeguarding children responsible for educating, advising and supporting staff, ensuring that appropriate local policies are in place and followed, and that accurate, timely recording of incidents are produced.

National policy guides practice, with a series of important documents making this explicit. The latest version of this is '*Working Together to Safeguard Children*' (Department for Education 2015). This emphasizes the importance of interagency and multiprofessional cooperation in keeping children safe. The named nurse will have a direct contact for the appropriate social worker in the local authority as well as the means to share information with the health visitor. There are explicit guidelines about when and how to share information, but they are facilitative rather than restricting.

Additional guidance for nurses is provided by the Royal College of Nursing (2014: 11) which reminds nurses that: 'A child's welfare is paramount in every respect, regardless of whether you feel sympathy for the parent or carer. You must always act on a child's behalf if you have concerns'. It is part of the nurse's role to place the child first, while also responding positively and respectfully to parents who may be under investigation for concerns about their child's welfare.

5 **What would a student nurse's role be?**

A Understandably, this can be a difficult issue for a student. However, senior nursing and medical staff will address the concerns in this case, and the student's role will be to record anything relevant that they might see or hear, to report promptly and discreetly to a senior member of staff, and to maintain a positive working relationship with the family in giving care as normal. Helpful, practical advice can be found in the report '*What to Do if You are Worried a Child is Being Abused*' (HM Government 2015).

Key points

- Careful attention must be paid to the handover from paramedics to emergency department staff, including the source of aspects of the history and their own observations in order to establish what has happened and therefore potential injuries to be considered.
- The role of the trauma team is central to positive outcomes for patients. The role of each professional in the trauma team contributes to timely identification and prioritization of problems, means of investigation and the optimum treatment plan.
- Nurses must always be vigilant for signs of potential child abuse, including aspects of the history, parental behaviour or the nature of injuries; knowing how to raise concerns and maintaining an ethical, professional approach.

REFERENCES

Department for Education (2015) *Working Together to Safeguard Children. A Guide to Interagency Working to Safeguard and Promote the Welfare of Children*. London: Department of Education. Available at: *https://www.gov.uk/government/publications/working-together-to-safeguard-children–2* (accessed 9 February 2016).

Evans SM, Murray A, Patrick I, Fitzgerald M, Smith S, Cameron P (2010) Clinical handover in the trauma setting: a qualitative study of paramedics and trauma team members. *Quality & Safety in Health Care* 19: e57 (DOI:10.1136/qshc.2009.039073). Available at: http://qualitysafety. bmj.com/content/early/2010/08/10/qshc.2009.039073.full (accessed 23 January 2016).

Greater Manchester Critical Care Institute (2013) *Paediatric Acute Illness Management (PaedAIM Course Manual)*. Available at: http://www.gmccsi.org.uk/aim/paediatric-aim (accessed 22 January 2016).

HM Government (2015) *What to Do if You're Worried a Child is Being Abused. Advice for Practitioners*. London: HM Government. Available at: https://www.gov.uk/government/uploads/system/ uploads/attachment_data/file/419604/What_to_do_if_you_re_worried_a_child_is_being_ abused.pdf (accessed 9 February 2016).

National Institute for Health and Care Excellence (2014) *Head Injury. Triage, Assessment, Investigation and Early Management of Head Injury in Children, Young People and Adults. NICE Clinical Guideline 176*. London: NICE. Available at: https://www.nice.org.uk/guidance/cg176 (accessed 23 January 2016).

Royal College of Nursing (2014) *Safeguarding Children and Young People – Every Nurse's Responsibility*. London: RCN. Available at: https://www2.rcn.org.uk/__data/assets/pdf_file/0004/ 78583/004542.pdf (accessed 23 January 2016).

Scottish Intercollegiate Guidelines Network (2009) *Early Management of Patients with a Head Injury (Guideline 110)*. Edinburgh: SIGN. Available at: http://www.sign.ac.uk/pdf/sign110.pdf (accessed 23 January 2016).

A child with a suspected diagnosis of typhoid fever following recent foreign travel

Rob Kennedy and Natalie Hill

Case outline

Dhruv, aged 4 years, returned from visiting his family in India following the celebrations of his sister's wedding. Dhruv is usually a playful, happy boy, but during the six week trip to Jaipur he started to complain of feeling generally unwell with 'tummy ache'. This resulted in him being unable to participate in the large family celebration as he progressed to develop profuse diarrhoea and lethargy the week prior to returning home.

Upon returning to the UK his mother, Kalarati, and father, Noor, were concerned that he was not getting any better despite their efforts to care for him. Profuse diarrhoea persisted along with general lethargy, a headache and persistent high temperature of 40°C. His five siblings did not demonstrate any signs of illness. Approximately 48 hours after returning home, Kalarati decided to take Dhruv to the local emergency department as he was still not feeling any better. A diagnosis of typhoid fever was made.

EPIDEMIOLOGY

Typhoid, also known as enteric fever, is generally a disease of countries with poor or inadequate sanitary standards, being waterborne (Connor and Schwartz 2005; Crump et al. 2004) and caused by ingestion of contaminated food or water that contains the bacterium *Salmonella typhi or paratyphi*. These bacterium species are known only to colonize humans with transmission being via the oral route following ingestion of contaminated food or water containing faeces (Sinha et al. 1999). It is estimated that one million or more organisms are needed to cause illness in healthy individuals, with the incubation time being up to three weeks (Clark et al. 2010). Diagnosis is determined as being either 'confirmed, probable or chronic' (World Health Organization [WHO] 2011, Table 9.1). Typhoid is highly contagious.

South Asia, parts of South-East Asia, the Middle East, Central and South America and Africa are known to be areas where the disease is endemic. In 2000, the global annual

Table 9.1 Standard case definitions and classifications of typhoid fever

Confirmed case

- A patient with persistent fever (38°C or more) lasting three or more days, with laboratory-confirmed S. typhi organisms (blood, bone marrow, bowel fluid)
- A clinical compatible case that is laboratory confirmed

Probable case

- A patient with persistent fever (38°C or more) lasting three or more days, with a positive sero-diagnosis or antigen detection test but no S. typhi isolation
- A clinical compatible case that is epidemiologically linked to a confirmed case in an outbreak

Chronic carrier

- An individual excreting S. typhi in the stool or urine for longer than one year after the onset of acute typhoid fever
- Short-term carriers also exist, but their epidemiological role is not as important as that of chronic carriers
- Some patients excreting S. typhi have no history of typhoid fever

Source: World Health Organization (2011).

incidence of the disease was estimated as being 2.17 million cases, with 216,510 deaths (Crump et al. 2004). Within the UK, cases of typhoid are usually imported diseases associated with foreign travel and related contact with those individuals (Figure 9.1). Occasional outbreaks of indigenous typhoid occur in the UK (Patel. et al 2010).

Areas where typhoid is endemic prove the most risky for foreign travel. In the Indian subcontinent where there is a high incidence of typhoid fever, Crump et al. (2004) consider that there are approximately 100 cases per 100,000 people for the general population and 1 to 10 per 100,000 journeys made by visiting travellers (Connor and Schwartz 2005; Mermin et al. 1998; Steinberg et al. 2004).

It is believed that all patients who contract typhoid fever with the bacterium strain *Salmonella typhi (S. typhi)* will excrete the organism for approximately 3 months following the episode of acute illness. Approximately 2–5 per cent of these individuals will become long-term carriers of the disease. Deaths from typhoid fever are now virtually unheard of in the UK. However, if typhoid fever is not treated, it is estimated that up to one in five people with the condition will die. Some of those who survive typhoid fever will have permanent physical or mental disabilities. See Table 9.2 for groups at higher risk of transmitting gastrointestinal pathogens.

In the UK, Public Health England reported 311 confirmed cases in 2014, which was reduced in comparison to 502 confirmed cases in 2006 (Public Health England 2015). Of all reported cases in 2006, 45.2 per cent were of the S. typhi strain, with 59.5 percent of cases in 2014 being of type S. paratyphi A. The strain S. paratyphi B is rarely reported, with only 117 being notified in the eight-year-period 2006–2014 (Public Health England 2015). The main cause of typhoid in all cases is directly linked to foreign travel, particularly in India, Pakistan, Bangladesh, Thailand, Bolivia, Philippines, Tanzania, South Africa, Cambodia, Nepal, Malaysia, Mozambique and Senegal (Public Health England 2015).

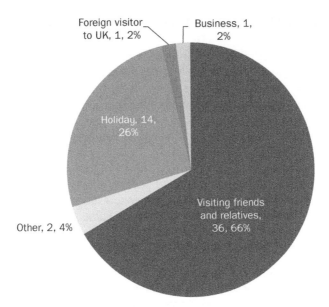

Figure 9.1 Laboratory confirmed cases of enteric fever in individuals that have travelled abroad (N = 54) by reason for travel in the second quarter of 2015

Source: adapted from Public Health England (2015).

Table 9.2 Groups at higher risk of transmitting gastrointestinal pathogens

Risk group	Description	Additional comments
Group A	Any person of doubtful personal hygiene or with unsatisfactory toilet, handwashing or hand drying facilities at home, work or school	Risk assessment should consider, for example, hygiene facilities at the workplace
Group B	All children aged 5 years old or under who attend school, preschool, nursery or other childcare or minding groups	Explore informal childcare arrangements
Group C	People whose work involves preparing or serving unwrapped food to be served raw or not subjected to further heating	Consider informal food handlers, e.g. someone who regularly helps to prepare buffets for a congregation
Group D	Clinical, social care or nursery staff who work with young children, the elderly, or other particularly vulnerable people, and whose activities increase the risk of transferring infection via the faeco-oral route. Such activities include helping with feeding or handling objects that could be transferred to the mouth	Someone may be an informal carer, e.g. caring for a chronically sick relative

Source: Public Health England (2012).

FORMAL DIAGNOSIS AND REPORTING

Diagnosis of enteric fever is governed by public health and WHO statutes within law. Salmonella isolates must be sent to the National Microbiology Reference Laboratory (NMRL) by law. Definitive diagnosis of enteric fever is by culture of the organism from the blood or faeces. It is possible to isolate the organisms within the blood earlier on in the disease process. Urine and faeces will have organisms present after approximately one week. The results of any culture are generally available 72 hours later (WHO 2003).

- Blood culture is usually positive in only 50 per cent of all cases.
- Stool culture is not usually positive during the acute illness phase of the disease.
- Bone-marrow cultures increase the diagnostic accuracy to about 80 per cent of cases, but this is invasive and can be painful.
- Blood and stool cultures are the most widely used (in combination).

1   **As the practitioner caring for Dhruv and his family, what do you believe are the public health impacts of the disease? Do you need to consider his parents and five siblings, too?**

Extra resource

To help with your answer, look at the Public Health England (2012) Typhoid and paratyphoid operational guidelines (see Figure 9.2).

(A) IMMEDIATE DIAGNOSIS AND TREATMENT

Upon clinical assessment, Dhruv demonstrates signs of being grossly dehydrated, reporting stomach cramps, appears deeply lethargic, has a reduced urine output and is anorexic. A stool sample is taken that demonstrates a positive result for *Salmonella enterica*, confirming the diagnosis of typhoid fever. Dhruv is treated immediately for dehydration, receiving intravenous fluids and antibiotics. You have learned about rehydration in earlier cases. Treatment should focus initially upon the clinical management of his immediate needs, and it can be seen in Table 9.1 that his symptoms fall into the 'confirmed case' section. He has an acute and uncomplicated episode of the disease that should be easily manageable.

It is explained to his parents that typhoid fever is a notifiable disease to Public Health England and highly contagious, although easily treated. For this reason, Dhruv needs to receive his initial hospital treatment in strict isolation until he has three negative stool samples and his clinical condition has improved.

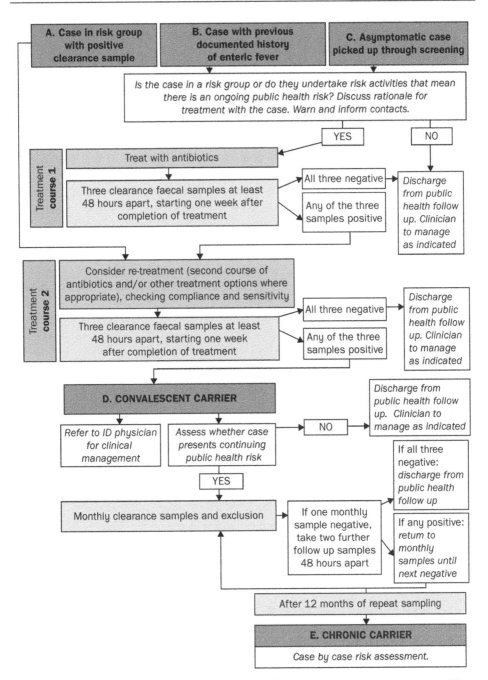

Figure 9.2 Public health management of cases with positive screening, clearance samples and those with previous documented history of enteric fever

Public Health Operational Guidelines for Enteric Fever V1.0 (Public Health England (2012).

MANAGEMENT OF MORE SEVERE CASES

Unfortunately, not all individuals are as lucky as Dhruv, and some have a particularly complicated disease process. Up to 10 per cent of patients develop life-threatening complications. In these cases, abdominal discomfort can lead to perforation of the peritoneal contents, peritonitis and severe sepsis (WHO 2003, 2011). Altered mental status and conscious level can be indicative of severe dehydration, but can also be signs of something far more serious, with typhoid meningitis, encephalomyelitis, Guillain–Barré syndrome, cranial or peripheral neuritis and psychosis all being reported (WHO 2003, 2011). Massive haemorrhage has been noted in cases of typhoid fever. Hepatitis, myocarditis, pneumonia, disseminated intravascular coagulopathy, thrombocytopenia and haemolytic uraemic syndrome are other potential effects (WHO 2003, 2011). Evidence suggests that in developing countries up to 15 per cent of typhoid patients die from prolonged, persistent fever for no clear reason.

Typhoid can be treated successfully using antibiotic regimens with supportive nursing and medical care. Evidence suggests, however, that certain strains of S. *typhi* have become increasingly resistant to antibiotic therapy. Threlfall and Ward (2001) consider that strains derived from South Asia are more likely to be resistant and thus impact upon the ability to treat successfully with traditional antibiotic regimens such as chloramphenicol, co-trimoxazole and amoxicillin (Bhutta et al. 1991). In resistant cases, the use of third-generation cephalosporins or azithromycin or ceftriaxone may be required (Threlfall and Ward 2001).

2   **As the nurse providing care to Dhruv, develop an infection control care plan that incorporates standard procedures and demonstrates why these are necessary. You will need to consider some of the following issues.**

- What are standard infection control precautions, and why are they necessary?
- When should standard infection control precautions be instigated?
- What are transmission-based precautions?
- What are your responsibilities towards yourself and your patients?

A   Dhruv's infection control care plan should be similar to the one in Table 9.3.

Standard infection prevention and control measures are an intrinsic part of any nurse's practice (National Patient Safety Agency [NPSA] 2004; Oughtibridge 2003; Siegel et al. 2007) and have been proven to reduce the use of antibiotic therapies in adults and children (House of Lords Select Committee on Science and Technology 1998; Millward et al. 1993). However, sometimes these measures are not sufficient in protecting the population from virulent infection, such as typhoid, and further transmission-based precautions need to be implemented (Health Protection Scotland [HPS] 2014). Transmission-based precautions can be defined as: 'a set of infection prevention and control measures that should be implemented when patients are known or suspected to be infected with an infectious agent. These should be implemented, as required, in addition to standard infection control precautions and are applicable in all care settings' (HPS 2014: p. 6).

Table 9.3 Infection control care plan

Nursing need	Therapeutic intervention
Dhruv has a diagnosis of typhoid and is required to be nursed in strict isolation	• Involve the hospital infection control team and inform them of a positive diagnosis • Isolate the patient in a single room with en-suite facilities to reduce cross-contamination • If en-suite is not available ensure access to own commode at all times • Place an isolation sign on the outside of the door to inform the requirement for isolation • If there are no single rooms available, contact a member of the infection control team for advice • Reinforce requirements for barrier nursing with the parents to support understanding and concordance with treatment plan
Dhruv should be cared for using strict hand hygiene to prevention cross-contamination	• Hand hygiene must be performed before and after contact with Dhruv or objects in the room • Soap and water or alcohol gel (if hands are visibly clean) can be used for hand decontamination • Gloves should be used to prevent hand contamination. After glove removal hands must be decontaminated • Ensure handwashing facilities are offered to the patient regularly, especially before eating and after using the toilet • Encourage parents to keep Dhruv's nails short and clean
Dhruv should be cared for wearing personal protective equipment (PPE)	• Wear plastic aprons and gloves for contact with Dhruv, the immediate patient environment and equipment • Visitors are not required to wear gloves and aprons
Decontamination of patient equipment	• When possible, equipment should be designated for Dhruv's own use and kept in the room • Equipment removed from the room must be cleaned with chlorine-based detergent • Patient crockery/cutlery should be removed from the room and washed in the normal way • Keep items/equipment to a minimum within the room • Equipment should be cleaned between and after use
Clinical waste disposal	• Dispose of all waste into clinical waste pedal bin inside room. When sack three-quarters full fasten securely • Label with ward ID

(Continued overleaf)

Table 9.3 *(Continued)*

Nursing need	Therapeutic intervention
Environmental cleaning	• To maintain confidentiality, advise domestic staff that the patient is being isolated • Floor, surfaces, sink, toilet etc. must be cleaned twice daily by domestic staff using chlorine-based detergent • Please refer to standard operating procedures twice daily clean of isolation rooms • Nursing staff are responsible for the cleaning of patient-related equipment twice daily using chlorine-based detergent • When room vacated nursing staff should clean patient-related equipment with chlorine-based detergent and remove it from the room. Domestic staff should then carry out a thorough terminal clean of the room. When dry, the room can be used. Please refer to standard operating procedures terminal clean of isolation room
Laundry	• All patients' linen should be changed on a daily basis. • Place used linen in alginate bag, then clear polythene bag, then into a white laundry bag • Clean linen to be taken into the room only when required. Do not store clean linen in room • Ensure the patient information leaflet 'Taking laundry home – information for carers' is provided if required
Dhruv should be cared for in isolation with limited visiting	• Dhruv should have age-appropriate care delivered for a 4-year-old in order to maintain well-being and to support cognitive developmental needs. Therapeutic play should be instigated. • Visitors do not have to wear PPE but must ensure they decontaminate their hands before and after leaving the room • Visitors should be discouraged from sitting on the patient's bed • Visitors report to nurse in charge before entering • Visitors are not required to wear gloves and aprons, but should wash their hands when leaving the room • Dhruv should only be removed from isolation when clinically stable and three negative stool specimens have been examined

Based upon guidance from NHS Greater Glasgow and Clyde (2015) http://www.nhsggc.org.uk/your-health/public-health/infection-prevention-and-control/

These precautions should be applied when caring for a patient that has an active infection. Typhoid is an example of this and in Dhruv's case his plan of care should reflect the requirement for standard and transmission-based precautions as there is a need to protect others. Other patients need to be protected by the prevention of 'contact transmission' (HPS 2014). As Dhruv will be infectious for prolonged periods of time, up to 3 months or more (Public Health England 2015), direct transmission of typhoid through contact, direct or indirect, is a possibility.

The most likely transmission route is via healthcare workers' hands if hand hygiene is not performed adequately or between engaging in direct care for more than one patient. Transmission from an infected, contaminated, colonized patient through touch can occur readily. Accordingly, effective handwashing and appropriate use of standard infection prevention and control measures (HPS 2014; Public Health England 2015; NPSA 2004; Siegel et al. 2007) are key to prevention of cross-contamination (Alspach 2008; WHO 2009).

Extra resource

See the particularly clear diagrams of effective hand decontamination (p.156) and of transmission of infection by touch (pp.15–19) in the WHO (2009) report at http://apps.who.int/iris/bitstream/10665/44102/1/9789241597906_eng.pdf

---

3 **What is the role of vaccination in preventing typhoid?**

A Vaccination has proven to be very successful in many parts of the world in adults, children and young people. Infants under 1 year should not be immunized. For those between 12 months and 2 years, immunization should only be considered if the risk of developing typhoid fever is considered very high. Vaccination should be avoided in the young child who is immunosuppressed (American Academy of Pediatrics 2012; Department of Health 2011).

Three types of vaccine are available internationally: polysaccharide vaccine; oral, live vaccine; and whole-cell inactivated vaccine. In the UK, the Vi polysaccharide vaccine is considered to be the most efficacious following evaluated field studies (Acharya et al 1987; Klugman et al. 1987, 1996). However, little data exists to support its efficacy and use in children aged less than 18 months (Cadoz 1998). The preferred route of administration is oral dosing with the fluoroquinolones: a family of broad spectrum, systemic antibacterial agents (Chinh and Parry 2000).

THE OUTLOOK FOR DHRUV

Of all patients with a diagnosis of typhoid fever, up to 5 per cent will become chronic carriers of the bacterium, harbouring *S. typhi* within their gall bladder. However, Dhruv should be expected to recover completely, with no persisting effects. Further public health advice will be provided for the family, in anticipation of further international travel, and efforts will be made to return Dhruv to his normal pattern of activity, including nursery or preparation for school.

Key points

- Air travel to all parts of the world presents risks of communicable diseases being imported and spread in countries where the disease is not normally found. Vigilance and thoughtful consideration of a history of travel to affected countries or zones should be part of the assessment process in cases with relevant symptoms.
- With adherence to clear infection control guidelines regarding isolation, management of infected materials, supervision of visitors, and monitoring for continued infection, it is possible to maintain normal nursing standards while protecting staff, visitors, and other patients from individuals with infectious diseases.
- Handwashing is of the utmost importance. Both practical handwashing technique and routines for when this should be undertaken are essential to effectiveness of infection control.

REFERENCES

Acharya IL, Lowe CU, Thapa R, et al. (1987) Prevention of typhoid fever in Nepal with the Vi capsular polysaccharide of *Salmonella typhi*. A preliminary report. *New England Journal of Medicine* 317: 1101–1104.

Alspach G (2008) Protecting your patients, colleagues, family, and yourself from infection: first wash. *Critical Care Nurse* 28(1): 7–12.

American Academy of Pediatrics (2012) Active and passive immunization., in LK Pickering, CJ Baker, DW Kimberlin, SS Long (eds) *Red Book: Report of the Committee on Infectious Diseases* (29th edn). Elk Grove Village, IL: American Academy of Pediatrics.

Bhutta ZA, Naqvi SH, Suria A (1991) Chloramphenicol therapy of typhoid fever and its relationship to hepatic dysfunction. *Journal of Tropical Pediatrics* 37: 320–332.

Cadoz M (1998) Potential and limitations of polysaccharide vaccines in infancy. *Vaccine* 16: 1391–1395.

Chinh N, Parry C (2000). A randomised controlled comparison of azithromycin and ofloxacin for multidrug-resistant and nalidixic acid resistant enteric fever. *Antimicrobial Agents and Chemotherapy* 44: 1855–1859.

Clark T, Daneshvar C, Pareek M, Perera N, Stephenson I (2010) Enteric fever in a UK regional infectious diseases unit: A 10 year retrospective review. *Journal of Infection* 60: 91–98.

Connor BA, Schwartz E (2005) Typhoid and paratyphoid fever in travellers. *Lancet Infectious Diseases* 5: 623–628.

Crump JA, Luby SP, Mintz ED (2004) The global burden of typhoid fever. *Bulletin of the World Health Organization* 82: 346–353.

Department of Health (2011) *Green Book: Immunisation against Infectious Disease* [updated 2011 March]. London: Department of Health.

Health Protection Scotland (2014) *National Infection Prevention and Control Manual*. Glasgow: HPS. Available at: http://www.documents.hps.scot.nhs.uk/hai/infection-control/ic-manual/ipcm-p-v2-3.pdf (accessed 23 January 2016).

House of Lords Select Committee on Science and Technology (1998) *Resistance to Antibiotics and Other Microbial Agents*. London: The Stationery Office.

Klugman KP, Gilbertson IT, Koornhof HJ, et al. (1987) Protective effect of Vi capsular polysaccharide vaccine against typhoid fever. *Lancet* 2(8569): 1165–1169.

Klugman KP, Koornhof HJ, Robbins JB, Le Cam NN (1996) Immunogenicity, efficacy and serological correlate of protection of Salmonella typhi Vi capsular polysaccharide vaccine three years after immunization. *Vaccine* 14: 435–438.

Mermin JH, Townes JM, Gerber M, Dolan N, Mintz ED, Tauxe RV (1998) Typhoid fever in the United States, 1985-1994. Changing risks of international travel and increasing antimicrobial resistance. *Archives of Internal Medicine* 158: 633–638.

Millward S, Barnett J, Thomlinson D (1993) A clinical infection control audit programme. Evaluation of a tool used by infection control nurses to monitor and assess effective staff training. *Journal of Hospital Infection* 24(3): 219–232.

National Patient Safety Agency (2004) *Clean Your Hands Campaign*. London: NHS England. Available at: http://www.npsa.nhs.uk/cleanyourhands/ (accessed 23 January 2016).

NHS Greater Glasgow and Clyde (2015) *Care Plans*. Glagow: NHSGGC. Availabe at http://www.nhsggc.org.uk/your-health/public-health/infection-prevention-and-control/care-plans/ (accessed 23 January 2016).

Oughtibridge D (2003) The modern matron. *Nursing Management* 10(2): 26–28.

Patel TA, Armstrong M, Morris-Jones SD, Wright SG, Doherty T (2010) Imported enteric fever: case series from the hospital for tropical diseases, London, United Kingdom. *American Journal of Tropical Medicine and Hygiene* 82(6): 1121–1126.

Public Health England (2012) *Public Health Operational Guidelines for Typhoid and Paratyphoid (Enteric Fever)*. London: PHE. Available at: https://www.gov.uk/government/uploads/system/uploads/attachment_data/file/355864/Public_Health_Operational_Guidelines_for_Enteric_Fever_v1.0_Feb_2012.pdf (accessed 23 January 2016).

Public Health England (2015) *Enteric Fever (Typhoid And Paratyphoid) England, Wales and Northern Ireland*: 2014. London: PHE. Available at: https://www.gov.uk/government/uploads/system/uploads/attachment_data/file/488395/Enteric_fever_annual_report_2014_FINAL_.pdf (accessed 9 February 2016).

Siegel JD, Rhinehart E, Jackson M, Chiarello L (2007) *Guideline for Isolation Precautions: Preventing Transmission of Infectious Agents in Healthcare Settings 2007*. Atlanta, GA: Centres for Disease Control and Prevention. Available at: http://www.cdc.gov/hicpac/pdf/isolation/Isolation2007.pdf (accessed 23 January 2016).

Sinha A, Sazawal S, Kumar R, et al. (1999) Typhoid fever in children aged less than 5 years. *Lancet* 354: 734–737.

Steinberg EB, Bishop R, Haber P, et al. (2004) Typhoid fever in travellers: who should be targeted for prevention? *Clinical Infectious Diseases* 39: 186–191.

Threlfall EJ, Ward LR (2001) Decreased susceptibility to ciprofloxacin in Salmonella enterica serotype typhi, United Kingdom. *Emerging Infectious Diseases* 7: 448–450.

World Health Organization (2003) *Background Document: The Diagnosis, Treatment and Prevention of Typhoid Fever*. Geneva: WHO.

World Health Organization (2009) *WHO Guidelines on Hand Hygiene in Health Care: First Global Patient Safety Challenge Clean Care is Safer Care*. Geneva: WHO. Available at: http://apps.who.int/iris/bitstream/10665/44102/1/9789241597906_eng.pdf (accessed 23 January 2016).

World Health Organization (2011) *Guidelines for the Management of Typhoid Fever*. Geneva: WHO. Available at: http://apps.who.int/medicinedocs/documents/s20994en/s20994en.pdf (accessed 23 January 2016).

CASE STUDY 10

Planned elective surgery for congenital spinal disorder: post-surgical care

Tony Long and Natalie Hill

Case outline

Maria, who is 13 years old, was diagnosed with congenital scoliosis when she was 11 following increasing concern about the prominence of ribs on one side and obviously uneven hips. The diagnosis was confirmed by x-ray and magnetic resonance imaging. Since the angle of curvature has increased to 47 degrees and is still worsening, the decision has been made to undertake surgery (insertion of a spinal rod) to correct the problem and prevent further worsening. Although this is major surgery, the operation is concluded without any undue problems, and Maria is transferred to the intensive care unit to recover.

THE NORMAL SPINE

In order to understand the problems presented in this case, it would be helpful to familiarize yourself with the normal shape of the spine. A life-size model is best for this, but many suitable diagrams are available in textbooks and on the internet.

Extra resource

See Disabled World (2016), for an example of a spine diagram: http://www.disabled-world.com/artman/publish/spine_picture.shtml

---

SCOLIOSIS

Congenital scoliosis is characterized by lateral curvature and rotation of the thoracic (chest) or lumber (lower back) spine caused by a defect in the formation of the spinal column. Although the vertebral abnormality develops before birth, clinical signs of

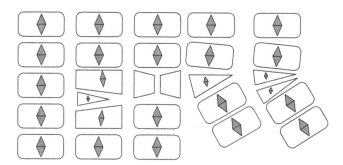

Figure 10.1 Variety of spinal deformities

deformity may not be evident until later in childhood as asymmetric growth occurs in the spinal column. A variety of vertebral malformations may exist: misshapen (wedge-shaped), half-formed (hemi-vertebrae) or un-segmented (failure to separate at either side) vertebrae may be present (Figure 10.1).

There are other forms of scoliosis (caused by other pathology or medical condition) that may develop in early childhood and not before birth, but in these cases there are no abnormal vertebrae. In about 80 per cent of all scoliosis cases there is no known cause. This is termed idiopathic scoliosis (Scoliosis Association UK 2013).

The displacement of the spine alters the spacing of the ribs, leads to a characteristic lump on the back, and often causes the scapula to be pulled out of alignment. The spine may be affected in more than one area, causing an S-shaped or irregular deformity. Two terms are important.

- **Kyphosis:** this describes the jutting out (backwards) of the upper (thoracic) part of the spine. Stiffness, restricted movement and back pain commonly develop. A smaller degree of thoracic kyphosis is normal.
- **Lordosis:** this is characterized by the forward deformity of the middle and lower (lumbar) regions of the spine. A degree of lumbar lordosis is normal.

Extra resource

The way in which such malformation is presented to patients and their families is important. See the information offered by Boston Children's Hospital (Centre for Young Women's Health 2013) for an example of this. http://youngwomenshealth.org/2013/10/31/scoliosis-and-spinal-deformities/

1 **If this is a congenital condition, why was Maria diagnosed so late?**

A Although the spinal malformations are present at birth in congenital scoliosis, this does not mean that there was spinal curvature at birth. Scoliosis (the twisting of the spine) does not develop until later in most cases – often not until adolescence. The defect in itself is rarely painful, so other signs have to develop before the condition becomes clinically obvious.

2 **Understanding the anatomy of the spine and the nearby organs is important when thinking about the impact of scoliosis and the effects of surgery. Where does the spinal cord lie?**

(a) In front of the vertebral bodies.
(b) Down the centre of the spinal column.
(c) Behind the vertebral bodies.

A The weight of the body is carried through the vertebral bodies – discs of bone behind which there is a natural space (the spinal canal or vertebral foramen) enclosed by the pedicles and lamina through which runs the spinal cord. The spinal cord runs behind the vertebral bodies.

OTHER PROBLEMS THAT MIGHT BE ASSOCIATED WITH SCOLIOSIS

The heart and the kidneys develop at the same time as the vertebrae, so anomalies in the cardiac vessels in the heart itself or in the kidneys or bladder can also occur. Problems may also be found with the oesophagus or the lungs, although less commonly.

Post-operative care

In immediate post-operative care, much depends upon the length of time taken to complete the operation (and therefore the length of the anaesthetic). Maria's operation lasted for almost 10 hours. She was taken to the paediatric intensive care unit from the operating theatre still intubated and ventilated. This continued until the following morning when she was extubated.

3 **Imagine yourself in Maria's place. Although there had been time and opportunity to prepare her for the surgery and to answer any questions or concerns, how might she feel physically and psychologically when she awakes from the sedation and over the next few days?**

4 **How would you implement pain management?**

A With such invasive surgery as this and a large wound, you should expect pain management to be a substantial part of the care plan, and a formal protocol should be followed. As with all children, guidance from the pain management team is vital. Both morphine and ketamine will be given for the first 48 hours, and sometimes an epidural block will be used, too. By the second post-operative day, it is usually possible to start reducing the dosage and strength of the analgesic drugs. Paracetamol would follow. Even at 13 years and following major surgery, Maria will benefit from distraction therapy from play specialists.

5 **What would you do to offer psychological support in regaining mobility?**

A Despite prior explanation, it is likely that Maria will be afraid to move or to cough, and generally will be anxious about her treatment and progress. The distraction therapy is also part of the effort to calm Maria and to enforce a little normality into a largely abnormal experience. Addressing her fears is important given the risks to her of immobility. Take a moment to think what these might be if you did not identify this earlier. Immobility coupled with fear of deep breathing or coughing poses a risk of chest infection, particularly after a long anaesthetic. Successful management of pain and thoughtful repetition of explanations about the need to move and become mobile as early as possible will encourage Maria to cooperate in efforts to achieve this. A potential reward for improved mobility is access to a normal toilet. It would be expected that Maria would be able to sit out of bed on her second post-operative day, gradually progressing to walking with support and then unsupported.

6 **How would these issues impact on skin integrity?**

A During surgery and for the period afterwards while her mobility is restricted, Maria is at risk of pressure sores, particularly with additional pressure points and following a long period of sedation. This is a good example of elements of care being interwoven. Without adequate pain relief she will be too sore to move. Without psychological support she will be afraid to move. So tissue viability rests not only on effective pressure area care techniques and aids, but also on other aspects of care.

7 **Why would management of fluid balance be important?**

A Prolonged major surgery of this nature implies significant blood loss during surgery as well as continued fluid loss into the wound area post-operatively. Some of this fluid will be lost through drains, and some will be effectively lost from the circulation into tissue around the wound although not externally from the body. Large volumes of intravenous fluid replacement will be required for the first 48 hours, including blood transfusion for some patients. Fortunately, Maria, as with most otherwise healthy teenagers, will tolerate a fairly low haemoglobin level. Many specialist centres will extract and store the patient's own blood weeks before surgery for autologous transfusion if required. Meticulous recording of fluid balance is required, which, together with routine blood sampling will guide fluid replacement.

8 **How would you deal with wound drains?**

A Parker et al. (2008) have shown that wound drains in general orthopaedic surgery are ineffective in reducing the incidence of haematoma or infection, so their use has been largely discontinued. If they are used, wound drains will be removed once drainage is minimal, and usually within 24 hours. Specific to this operation, however, a spinal chest drain will have been inserted, and this will be removed after 24 hours. A waterproof dressing will have been applied over subcutaneous soluble sutures, so showering will be allowed. Other than keeping the wound socially clean (that is, at a normal level of cleanliness rather than aseptic practice), no other treatment should be required.

9   **What sort of monitoring will be needed?**

A   Arterial and central venous pressure monitoring will be maintained for the first 48 hours, and neurological observation of sensation in the limbs will be recorded hourly for the first 24 hours, then four-hourly for the next 48 hours, and then at a decreasing frequency until Maria is moving around independently.

10   **What are the infection risks?**

A   As with any patient who has been subjected to a long period of anaesthesia followed by restricted mobility, there are risks of chest infection, infection around the urinary catheter or central venous catheter, and in the wound. Antibiotic treatment should not be routine but reserved for cases where infection is apparent. The physiotherapist will help to keep Maria's chest clear.

11   **Should eating be a problem?**

A   Although nausea can be problematic after this surgery, there is no other physiological barrier to Maria recommencing a normal diet.

12   **What would you do to support Maria's family and engage them in her care?**

A   Family responses to the surgery vary, with some families encouraging increased mobility and others adding another psychological barrier to this. Tactful explanation both before and after the surgery of how families can help and the need to trust the staff may promote a supportive, positive presence. Maria's parents also require psychological support given the enormity of the experience for them and their daughter.

13   **What will be the plan for Maria's discharge home?**

A   Most patients will remain in the hospital for about 3–6 days after surgery. Once pain is well-controlled, when Maria is able to eat and drink without nausea, and when she can walk around, she can expect to go home. Her family will have been instructed on what problems to look for, as well as how to manage her diet and medications prior to discharge.

The family will be urged to contact the surgical team immediately and directly if any of the following are experienced:

- fever, chills, redness, warmth, or foul smell from the surgical site
- increase in pain that is not controlled with medications
- numbness, tingling, or weakness in the arms or legs
- change in bowel or bladder control.

Maria will not be able to return to school for six weeks after surgery. Home tuition will be arranged through her school. An outpatient clinic appointment will be made for six weeks after surgery.

THE LONG-TERM OUTLOOK

Since treatment has improved drastically, together with supportive therapy, the outlook should be encouraging for Maria. Kepler et al. (2012) found that most adolescents who had undergone fusion surgery for idiopathic scoliosis experienced positive outcomes. Some degree of further degeneration of vertebrae beyond the location of fusion might occur, but usually remained 'clinically silent' – asymptomatic. Research from Denmark suggests that health-related quality of life for people who were treated for scoliosis in adolescence remained within the range of normal for the general population 25 years after surgery with Harrington Rod or fusion, and no deterioration was found in deformity (Simony et al. 2015).

Extra resource

Round this case off by watching 'Rachel's story' of living with scoliosis and the treatment that she had over the years (NHS Choices 2015): http://www.nhs.uk/conditions/scoliosis/Pages/Introduction.aspx

---

Key points

- Clear understanding of anatomy (in three dimensions) and organs that could be implicated by deformity or disease is important in clinical practice. In Maria's condition, curvature of the spine occurs in two planes and at different levels, squashing organs and altering posture.
- Even with such extensive surgery, post-operative nursing care is structured by addressing problems (actual or potential), and including both psychological and physical aspects of need. Tailoring the plan to the patient's age, level of development and personal concerns is always central.
- You should be clear about the long-term outlook for patients after major surgery, being ready to respond to the family's worries, but also encouraging restoration of normal activity and life. This means being aware of the evidence base for prognosis and sources of ongoing support.

REFERENCES

Centre for Young Women's Health (2013) *Scoliosis and Spinal Deformities*. Boston, MA: Boston Children's Hospital. Available at: http://youngwomenshealth.org/2013/10/31/scoliosis-and-spinal-deformities/ (accessed 23 January 2016).

Disabled World (2016) *Human Spinal Cord and Spine Pictures Showing C1 to S5 Vertebra*. Available at: http://www.disabled-world.com/artman/publish/spine_picture.shtml (accessed 23 January 2016).

Kepler CK, Meredith DS, Green DW, Widmann RF (2012) Long-term outcomes after posterior spine fusion for adolescent idiopathic scoliosis. *Current Opinion in Pediatrics* 24(1): 68–75 (DOI: 10.1097/MOP.0b013e32834ec982).

NHS Choices (2015) Scoliosis: *Rachel's Story*. Available at: http://www.nhs.uk/conditions/scoliosis/Pages/Introduction.aspx (accessed 23 January 2016).

Parker MJ, Livingstone V, Clifton R, McKee A (2008) Closed suction surgical wound drainage after orthopaedic surgery. *Cochrane Database of Systematic Reviews* Jul 18, (3): CD001825. Available at http://onlinelibrary.wiley.com/doi/10.1002/14651858.CD001825.pub2/pdf (accessed 23 January 2016).

Scoliosis Association UK (2013) *Congenital Scoliosis.* London: Scoliosis Association UK. Available at: http://www.sauk.org.uk/about-scoliosis/congenital-scoliosis.html (accessed 23 January 2016).

Simony A, Hansen EJ, Carreon LY, Christensen SB, Andersen MO (2015) Health-related quality-of-life in adolescent idiopathic scoliosis patients 25 years after treatment. *Scoliosis* 10: 22 (DOI 10.1186/s13013-015-0045-8). Available at: http://www.scoliosisjournal.com/content/10/1/22 (accessed 23 January 2016).

PART 4
Trauma

CASE STUDY 11

A car accident in which the mother has been killed and the family injured

Tony Long, Sue Rothwell and Lindsay Sykes

Case outline

The Krakauer family has been involved in a road traffic collision while stationery at traffic lights. The mother, Vanessa, was driving and has sustained direct impact injuries, receiving resuscitation and immediate trauma treatment at the scene while being freed from the wreckage. Her injuries are non-survivable, and she dies soon after arriving at the accident and emergency (A&E) department. Her husband, Kris, and two children, Elise aged 4 and Martha aged 6, are all injured but not severely. Contact is made with Kris's brother who comes to the hospital to support the family.

This is a scenario that many students will dread, but it is thankfully rare and one that even specialist emergency department nurses would not expect to see more than once or twice in many years of practice. You should remember that in such situations the expertise of senior nurses and other staff will be brought to bear, and your own role will be to provide normal care, to reinforce messages that are instigated by senior staff, and to learn personally and professionally from the experience.

IMMEDIATE TREATMENT FOR KRIS AND THE CHILDREN

The move towards separate emergency departments for children or at least a separate area within a single department has been a major improvement in the experience for children (Royal College of Paediatrics and Child Health 2012). However, in unusual cases such as this in which adults and children are both affected by an incident, additional problems arise. Although attempts are made to keep children and parents together, the condition of the patients involved and the availability of dual trained nurses (adult and child) on duty have to be taken into account. In a large treatment centre it is likely that medical and nursing expertise in both adult and child health nursing will be available, but this may not be the case in a smaller hospital.

When children are involved in a road traffic collision that has involved a fatality they must be treated as a potential major trauma case. If a collision has been so severe that any occupant has been killed, the possibility of serious injury from the impact on other occupants of the same vehicle, even if not immediately apparent, must be investigated. You have already read about ABCDE (Airway, Breathing, Circulation, Disability, Exposure) assessment in Case 5, and MIST (Mechanism of the injury; Injuries sustained; Signs and symptoms; and Treatment) and AVPU (Alert, Voice, Pain, Unresponsive) in Case 8. The assessment is completed as quickly as possible to allow Elise and Martha to receive treatment and be comforted by their father. A nurse is allocated to each child for emotional support as well as physical nursing care during this process, talking to them and reassuring them.

THE ROLE OF HEALTH PLAY SPECIALISTS

Kris knows that Vanessa is dead but is unsure and worried about how and when to tell the children. Finding privacy and time to talk to Kris separately about what needs to be done is important, so distracting the children for a while allows time for the doctor who took responsibility for Vanessa's care to confirm the situation and to answer any immediate questions that Kris might have. Qualified health play specialists can help to normalize the emergency department environment, providing age- and need-appropriate distraction and play both to help the children to express their fears and desires, and to provide the opportunity for staff to help Kris with his own anguish and with preparing himself to talk to Martha and Elise about their mother (Tonkin 2014). Such information and insights as are elicited by play workers are passed on to the rest of the healthcare team to inform approaches and responses to the children.

1   **Taking into account the ages of the children as well as the treatment environment, what sort of games, pastimes or activities might be suitable to offer Martha and Elise?**

A   At 4 and 6 years old, the girls will enjoy creative activities, particularly activities that result in a product, that is, something that they have created. This could involve drawing or sticking. Alternatively, simple construction toys with which to make a model of an animal or a house, for example, would be suitable. Imaginative play using characters from children's television programmes would be welcomed, as would simple problem-solving such as jigsaws (12–20 pieces). Play specialists are expert at identifying potential uses for immediately available materials. Whenever you have the opportunity, ask why particular toys or activities have been chosen and add this new understanding to your own toolbox of strategies for working with children. The same approach can be used after children have been told of the death of someone special. See the booklet for children by Child Bereavement UK (2015).

VANESSA'S DEATH

Unless you have had personal experience of a similar bereavement, you may have little idea of the issues that need to be addressed when a patient dies in the hospital A&E department.

Legal requirements

Under the law, the death must be reported to the Coroner by the attending doctor. Specific reasons for reporting are provided:

- cause of death is unknown
- death was violent or unnatural
- death was sudden and unexplained
- person who died was not visited by a medical practitioner during their final illness
- medical certificate is not available
- person who died was not seen by the doctor who signed the medical certificate within 14 days before death or after they died
- death occurred during an operation or before the person came out of anaesthetic
- medical certificate suggests the death may have been caused by an industrial disease or industrial poisoning (HM Government 2015).

In this case, the death was violent and unnatural. Although the trauma team will have a clear idea of the cause of death from the injuries that were sustained, a Coroner's post-mortem will be required, in this case probably to be carried out at the hospital. The next of kin has no choice about this, but if they wish they can be informed of the date of the post-mortem examination. A post-mortem can be an additional source of anguish for a family, but gentle explanation of the need to confirm the precise cause of death, to establish the legal context of the case and to identify additional learning for medical teams can help with acceptance of the situation.

In cases of a violent or unnatural death the Coroner must hold an inquest. Further explanation of the reason for this and its format will be provided to the family. Most people will have little idea of the process of gaining a death certificate, registering the death or gaining permission to deal with the estate of the deceased.

> ### Extra resource
>
> Read the short but especially clear explanation for families provided by the Government (HM Government 2015).

THE ROLE OF THE FAMILY SUPPORT DEPARTMENT

Every hospital will have some form of organized family support, perhaps as separate teams for adult bereavement and child bereavement, although all will apply a similar approach. The role of the family support service is crucial in supporting families (adults and children) through the emotional turmoil and confusing practicalities of dealing with bereavement. Staff from this department will undertake most of this legal and practical aspect of guidance for family members in addition to providing emotional support. If you have the opportunity to be present and to observe them at their work, it would be a valuable learning experience.

2 Think for a moment about how you would prepare for a discussion with children about the death of a parent and how the discussion might be conducted. This will not be your role as a student, of course, but you may need to repeat the approach and messages as you provide care afterwards.

A Whenever it is possible, it is preferable for a parent or other family member to break the news to children. In this case, either Kris or his brother (unless another family member arrives soon) will need to do this. Even with training and experience, breaking such bad news can be a difficult task for any professional (Shoenberger et al. 2013). The issue will be discussed first with Kris, perhaps supported by his brother. Kris will be reassured that staff will stay with them while they tell Martha and Elise, and that they will help to comfort the children afterwards, too.

Winston's Wish (2015) offers advice to parents in plain terms about how to talk to children when someone has died, acknowledging that it is one of the hardest tasks that a parent may have. It is recommended that the conversation should be couched in age-appropriate language (as you would expect), but also that the messages should be truthful, direct and unambiguous. This may seem harsh, but see what Winston's Wish has to say about this, following feedback from children, and the guidance from Child Bereavement UK (2010).

> Younger children may be confused by some of the everyday expressions that people use when someone dies, such as describing the person as 'lost', 'gone' or 'passed away'. It is best to keep language simple and direct. Saying that someone has 'died' or is 'dead' is honest, helps to avoid confusion, and encourages acceptance.
>
> (Winston's Wish 2015)

Activity

Check out how children have responded to metaphorical or imprecise language at the Winston's Wish website. This is particularly convincing evidence that rather than being unfeeling and unnecessarily cruel, a direct, plain-English approach is best for children.

---

3 How might Martha and Elise understand and react to the news? Think about their age and stage of development. How would they understand the world?

A At 4 years of age, Elise may not understand what death means or grasp the permanent nature of death. Abstract thought is not yet developed. She will probably be aware that her father is sad and upset, and she may be desperate to see her mother again. If you are aware of attachment theory you might see how this could be applied to understand the perspective that Elise will have. At this age, children sometimes worry that something that they have done might be responsible for what has happened. You can expect Elise to react in many different ways, including failing to see any reason to be upset, and expecting to carry on as normal.

Being a little older, Martha is likely to have more notion of the meaning of death (perhaps from pets dying) and its permanence. Attending school acts to widen the breadth of a child's contacts and, therefore, of life stories from other children who have experienced a bereavement. Children of her age will often ask many questions about intricate details of why someone has died, associated events, arrangements and future issues. It is common for further questions to arise after a period of thought and reflection. This greater understanding may well lead to more explicit shows of emotion and distress. Allowing Martha to cry and express her feelings is important, although a common reaction is to try to cheer children up without allowing the flood of emotion to be released or to express an expectation that they will be brave and stop crying.

Activity

Read about children's reactions to death at different ages at the Cruse Bereavement Care website (www.cruse.org.uk/).

4 **What continuing support could be provided for the children from their father?**

A Kris and his family will benefit from advice that continuing to talk about Vanessa to the children, to remember shared experiences, answering more questions and agreeing to move on together as and when they can will help to support the children through their process of grieving and coming to terms with their new situation. One of their greatest fears that children express is that they will be unable to remember the parent or relative who has died (Winston's Wish 2015). A standard, but particularly effective strategy to adopt when children ask questions that might indicate that they are worrying is to reflect the question back by asking what they think. Then the child's response may elucidate what they are in fact thinking or worrying about, allowing for a better response to build from the conversation.

5 **What is the student nurse's role?**

A Once Kris and his brother have had the meeting with staff and then been helped to talk to Martha and Elise, a staff handover is completed so that all those who may become engaged with the family are aware of what has been said and the explanations that were offered to the children. This facilitates consistency in approach by the whole team. As a student you will have this same information, so if you find yourself looking after one of the children and they seek more information, you will be able to reinforce the messages that have been introduced with confidence and sincerity. If additional issues arise, it would be appropriate to respond that you will find out or ask someone who knows more to speak to the child.

STAFF NEED SUPPORT, TOO

It takes little imagination to see that this scenario would be distressing for staff and students. Mutual support and the opportunity to talk about the experience, releasing emotions in a safe, controlled setting are important aspects of helping all involved to put the situation in perspective and to reflect upon how the episode has affected them personally.

ONGOING CARE

Kris and his brother will disseminate the sad news through the family network. The approach taken to considering how to manage the long-term change for children is often that of 'the new normal'. Life will not be the same without Vanessa, but a new state of normality will develop as Kris and the children start gradually to carry on with life. For the children, support at school and nursery is important, so ensuring that staff at these establishments are aware of the family's changed situation is important.

Child Bereavement UK (2011a) has specific guidance on supporting younger children. Once Upon a Smile (2015), a charity in Manchester, offers support as aftercare to parents and children who have suffered the death of a family member. This support includes financial assistance, respite breaks for parents who have lost a partner or children who have lost a parent and bereavement support groups for children. Such groups tend to be local, so you could search to see what is available in your own region. Winston's Wish also provides support groups for children, a helpline, and a support website. There is more guidance again from Child Bereavement UK (2011b) on how adults can support bereaved children.

Key points

- Dealing with traumatic and unexpected sudden death can be challenging both practically and emotionally; especially so when children are involved. However, senior staff will lead the response, keeping others informed so that they can maintain the same approach in a supporting role.
- Even though patients may seem to be suffering only minor injuries, it is essential that normal assessment and treatment are provided, without distraction in clinical judgement by the emotional turmoil of the situation. If an incident is so severe that anyone is killed, the trauma team must start by suspecting the possibility of more serious injury to others.
- In any scenario in which caring staff are likely to be traumatized by their presence or participation (however experienced or senior), post-incident debriefing is a vital strategy to ensure that they receive support. Caring for carers is vital.

REFERENCES

Child Bereavement UK (2010) *Explaining to a Child that Someone has Died*. Saunderton: Child Bereavement UK. Available at: http://www.childbereavementuk.org/files/5614/0117/9770/Explaining_to_young_children_that_someone_has_died.pdf (accessed 24 January 2016).

Child Bereavement UK (2011a) *Supporting Bereaved Children Under 5 Years of Age*. Saunderton: Child Bereavement UK. Available at: http://www.childbereavementuk.org/files/3214/0117/8931/Supporting_bereaved_children_under_5.pdf (accessed 24 January 2016).

Child Bereavement UK (2011b) *What Helps Grieving Children and Young People*. Saunderton: Child Bereavement UK. Available at: http://www.childbereavementuk.org/files/2314/0117/9138/What_helps_grieving_children_and_young_people.pdf (accessed 24 January 2016).

Child Bereavement UK (2015) *When Someone Special has Died*. Saunderton: Child Bereavement UK. Available at: http://www.childbereavementuk.org/files/8114/0868/5880/Under_7s_A4.pdf (accessed 24 January 2016).

Cruse Bereavement Care (2015) *Children's Understanding of Death*. Richmond: Cruse Bereavement Care. Available at: http://www.cruse.org.uk/Children/children-understanding-death (accessed 24 January 2016).

HM Government (2015) *What to Do After Someone Dies*. London: HM Government. Available at: https://www.gov.uk/after-a-death/when-a-death-is-reported-to-a-coroner (accessed 24 January 2016).

Once Upon a Smile (2015) *How Do We Help?* Manchester: Once Upon a Smile. Available at: http://www.onceuponasmile.org.uk/what-we-do/ (accessed 24 January 2016).

Royal College of Paediatrics and Child Health (2012) *Standards for Children and Young People in Emergency Care Settings*. London: RCPCH. Available at:http://www.rcpch.ac.uk/sites/default/files/page/Intercollegiate%20Emegency%20Standards%202012%20FINAL%20WEB.pdf (accessed 24 January 2016).

Shoenberger JM, Yeghiazarian S, Rios C, Henderson SO (2013) Death Notification in the Emergency Department: Survivors and Physicians. *Western Journal of Emergency Medicine* 14(2): 181–185 (DOI: 10.5811/westjem.2012.10.14193). Available at: http://www.ncbi.nlm.nih.gov/pmc/articles/PMC3628479/ (accessed 24 January 2016).

Tonkin A (2014) The Provision of Play in Health Service Delivery. Fulfilling Children's Rights under Article 31 of the United Nations Convention on the Rights of the Child. Cambridge: NAHPS. Available at: http://nahps.org.uk/uploads/Final_full_report_NAHPS_.pdf (accessed 24 January 2016).

Winston's Wish (2015) *Talking About Death*. Cheltenham: Winston's Wish. Available at: http://www.winstonswish.org.uk/talking-about-death/ (accessed 24 January 2016).

CASE STUDY 12

An 11-year-old child with learning disability who steps into scalding bath water

Rob Kennedy

Case outline

David, aged 11 years, is admitted directly to the burns unit with burns to both of his feet, lower legs and buttocks. These occurred when David and his younger sister were playing while their mother was filling the bath with hot water. While his mother was distracted, David climbed onto the bath and fell into the scalding water. David has limited communication skills as a consequence of his autism. David was found to have approximately 11 per cent total body surface area burns.

1 **What do you think are the main issues to be addressed for David and his family? (Consider life threatening situations, comfort and psychological care.)**

A **IMMEDIATE BURN ASSESSMENT**

To ascertain the extent and severity of David's burn injuries, an immediate assessment of the total body surface area (TBSA) that is injured needs to be calculated. This will determine the surface area involved, but not the depth of the burn injury. In general, mortality rates rise with burn injuries that have greater TBSA and that are deep in very young or elderly patients.

In order to determine the surface area involved, David's burn injury is mapped upon a Lund and Browder chart (Lund and Browder 1944; Herndon 2013). This chart is divided into body surface areas both anteriorly and posteriorly and is extremely accurate in helping practitioners in calculating burn injury extent in children as it takes into account the changes in body surface proportions with growth and development over time. In children, a burn of 10 per cent TBSA or greater is generally considered to be a large burn. You can view a paediatric version of the Lund and Browder chart in the North West Children's Major Trauma Network's clinical guidelines 2015 (p. 79). There will also be copies in accident and emergency (A&E) departments and wards that deal with trauma cases where you might work.

RESUSCITATION

The second priority in David's care is fluid resuscitation. If adequate resuscitation is not initiated, cardiac output may decrease resulting in poor perfusion, organ dysfunction or death. For patients that receive adequate fluid resuscitation, cardiac output usually returns to normal within 24 to 36 hours following the burn injury. David's vital signs, level of consciousness, urine specific gravity, urine output and peripheral capillary refill are all parameters that determine adequate resuscitation. Shock is treated initially with 20 ml/kg of isotonic normal saline (0.9 per cent) or Hartmann's solution. The excessive fluid loss from the burn wound is replaced and calculated using the Parkland formula.

The Parkland formula uses Hartmann's solution, a crystalloid solution that can help to correct metabolic acidosis, as the lactate that is present in the Hartmann's solution is rapidly metabolized into bicarbonate (Herndon 2013).

3 x (weight in kg) x (TBSA burn) = 24 hour fluid replacement requirement

---

Calculation exercise

Using the above calculation, what are David's fluid requirements for 24 hours if he weighs 55 kg?
  The answer is given at the end of this case on p. 101.

It is extremely important to maintain an accurate record of all fluid input and output. David's condition will be monitored continuously, especially fluid balance, heart rate, respiration and blood pressure, which are good indicators of whether hypovolaemia is present. Additionally. blood samples will be taken at regular intervals to assess the packed cell volume/haematocrit (PCV/HCT), which will demonstrate the effectiveness of his overall fluid replacement. The amount of fluid given may be altered as indicated by these factors.

David will require maintenance fluid to counter metabolic loss in addition to the Parkland fluid resuscitation formula; this is calculated as below. Although this may be given intravenously at first, over time it should be reduced as he tolerates more orally. Sodium chloride 0.45 per cent and dextrose 5 per cent are usually used to provide the maintenance fluid required for children who have sustained burns. The amount to be given for each 24-hour period is calculated based upon the child's weight, as per the weight ranges that follow.

- Up to 10 kg = 100 ml/kg.
- 10–20 kg = 50 ml/kg (+ 1000 ml for first 10 kg).
- Over 20 kg = 20 ml/kg (+ 1500 ml for first 20 kg).

2 **What needs to be considered in terms of pain management?**

A It is generally accepted that all burn injuries are extremely painful. David will require carefully managed and adequate pain relief. The assessment of his pain should be performed using an appropriate tool taking into account David's age, developmental stage and also the impact of his diagnosis of autism. A suitable tool may include the Wong-Baker Faces Pain Rating Scale (2015): an easy to use, visual analogue scale that can be understood by a wide range of children in many different clinical situations.

Activity

Try a quick internet search for 'visual analogue scale pain' to see the wide variety of such scales that may be used.

A systematic review comparing the quality and effectiveness of various scales showed that there is little reason to choose one rather than another (Tomlinson et al. 2010). However, care must be taken with interpretation. For example, a child need not be crying to be in pain, and being sad will not always equate to being in pain. A child who experiences difficulty in understanding and expressing emotion might not recognize the significance of the different face types. Similarly, adult interpretations of colour (red as equating to burning or pain, for example) might not correlate well with children's perceptions of the same colours. Young children may not appreciate the impact of numbers, while being higher or lower on a ladder (as used in several versions of visual analogue pain scales) may mean nothing or have widely varying understanding for different children. Nevertheless, used with caution and skill both in communicating with children and interpreting their responses, such pain scales are a useful aid for gauging progress in pain management. The skills of communicating with children, including those who experience difficulty in this area for various reasons are considered at length by Kennedy and Binns (2014) and by Smith and Atkinson (2012).

Due to the extent of his burns David will require an intravenous infusion of morphine or Fentanyl to manage his pain. In addition, to reduce inflammation, ibuprofen or diclofenac may be used as they will also have an antipyretic effect. David would have supplementary doses of analgesic and sedative prior to cleaning and dressing of his burn wounds (National Institute for Health and Care Excellence [NICE] 2010: pp. 68–69).

3   **What about psychological aspects of David's care?**

A   It is important for all children and young people in hospital to have familiar faces present to reduce the impact of separation anxiety and promote effective communication; therefore it is appropriate for David to have his parents present during cannulation and other clinical procedures (Piira et al. 2005). David has a learning disability, and this needs to be taken into account, preferably through discussion and advice from his family. Whatever the degree of disability, nurses should recognize David's normal abilities first, find ways to accommodate his disability, and simply treat him individually as with any other patient. With positive action, a supportive environment and willingness on the part of health professionals to learn both from and about a patient with learning disability, the impact and disruption of hospitalization can be minimized. There is no reason why, with professional support and management of specific interests and needs, that David's process of learning and development should not continue in the acute hospital setting. Indeed, it is a right of all people with any disability to receive as good a service as anyone else receives (Michael 2008).

To gain a greater understanding of David's very specific and individual needs, an indepth assessment should be undertaken as part of the admission process. This should be in partnership with David (if possible) and his family (Pratt et al. 2012). This assessment highlights his essential, individualized needs. Used in conjunction with other communication strategies, nurses can be guided by this information, directing them to the best approaches to care for David that meet his needs through adaptations to their own clinical practice and the unusual environment in which David finds himself (Kennedy and Binns 2014; Miller and Aitken 2003).

David's mother (and indeed his sister) may feel some guilt as a result of David's injury. It will help assuage these feelings if the mother is allowed to express such feelings fully in a supportive environment and also continue to provide care for her son. Family counselling and psychological support should be offered.

4   How is burn depth assessment undertaken?

A   David has already had the extent of his burns quickly calculated as 11 per cent TBSA. The next stage in his immediate treatment is to ascertain the depth of his burn injuries. In order to achieve this safely and with minimal distress and anxiety to David, he will have received opiates as analgesia and an anxiolytic as sedation.

Assessment of depth is determined by the extent to which the heat from the hot water in the bath tub has caused tissue damage. Burn injuries cause coagulative necrosis of tissue, whereby the heat from the burning substance causes the blood within vessels to coagulate (clot) leading to cell rupture and death (Herndon 2013; Monstrey et al. 2008). As practitioners assessing burn wounds, this can be demonstrated by varying colours (indicated by blood flow) that determine the depth of injury through the three layers of skin.

The skin of a child is much thinner than in an adult and consequently burn injuries cause more damage to the child. The skin is the largest organ of the body and consists of three layers: epidermis, dermis and subcutaneous tissues. The epidermis functions to protect the skin from organisms. It contains a superficial layer called the stratum corneum. The stratum corneum prevents water and electrolyte loss, and if the epidermis is destroyed insensible heat loss from the body will increase, leading to hypothermia.

Extra resources

At this point it would help you to review the diagram of the skin in the Royal Manchester Children's Hospital leaflet 'Returning to school following a burn injury: a guide for school staff' (2013).

The next layer, the dermis, is thicker and makes up a large percentage of the skin, containing a large proportion of essential connective tissue, nerve endings, blood vessels, hair follicles, lymph spaces, sebaceous glands and sweat glands. If this area is damaged through burn injury or trauma the skin cannot regenerate or heal spontaneously as well as a burn to the epidermal layer.

The deepest layer consists of the subcutaneous tissue, which contains collagen and adipose (fatty) tissue. It is unusual but sometimes when this area is burned, exposure to bones, tendons and muscle may occur. With the loss of the protective barrier, the body is exposed to severe infections entering the wound. Wound healing will vary according to the severity of the burn. Burns are classified as superficial, superficial/partial, dermal and deep dermal/full-thickness burns. Erythema is never calculated as part of the TBSA of a burn injury.

SUPERFICIAL BURN

Superficial burns involve only the superficial epidermis. They are erythematous, very painful, but cause few systemic effects and only minimal tissue damage. The burn blanches to touch. An example of a superficial burn is sunburn. Healing occurs within three to five days as the epithelium peels away from the healed tissue that is below it.

PARTIAL-THICKNESS BURN

Partial-thickness burns involve the dermis. A classic sign of a partial-thickness burn is blistering. Minor partial-thickness burns involve the epidermis and the upper layers of the dermis. These burns are erythematous, very painful and deep and weeping blisters are present. When the blisters rupture, they are extremely painful to touch and are bright red in colour. Healing usually takes 10 to 21 days with minimal scarring. With a deep partial-thickness burn the epidermis is destroyed together with most of the dermis. It may blister, and is mostly dark red to pale in colour. The burn may blanch slowly to touch. Most children complain of discomfort rather than pain. Deep partial-thickness burns are whitish, soft and sensitive to pressure. Skin grafting is often required.

FULL-THICKNESS BURN

In a full-thickness burn, all of the layers of skin are destroyed. Full-thickness burns are dry, tough and leathery. They can be white, tan, brown or black (charred) in colour. The burn does not blanch to touch and the patient has no sensation in the burned area because of cellular nerve damage. A full-thickness burn may also involve muscle, fascia, bones and other deep structures.

Extra resources

You can see colour images of different thickness burns at the Forensicmed website (Forensic Medicine for Medical Students, 2015).

5 **What factors are considered in dressing the burns?**

A Dressing a burn wound becomes more complicated with increasing TBSA, and with injury depth and position. David's burns were 11 per cent TBSA and of superficial to partial thickness on his feet, lower legs and buttocks. The location of his injuries may impact upon his mobility and independence, and to help overcome this, assessment of functional mobility would involve other multidisciplinary-team members (Bosworth Bousfield 2002). A physiotherapists and an occupational therapist would participate in the dressing of the burn injuries in order to ensure correct anatomical positioning of his legs so as to optimize mobility and prevent contracture formation. David's burn wounds should heal within 10 to 21 days, assuming that optimal nutrition, fluid management and pain relief are achieved and that no infection develops.

Burn wounds are dressed as determined by the majority depth of the wound and the desired effect of the dressing product used. A multitude of dressing products are available for use. David's wounds will be dressed with a mixture of Betadine® and Biobrane®. Both types of dressing are applied only to the wound bed following thorough cleaning with simple baby soap and showering to rinse away any wound debris and contaminants. Microbiology wound swabs will be taken then to determine any bacterial contaminants that might indicate the need for a different dressing.

Betadine Ointment (povidone iodine) belongs to a class of antiseptics known as iodophores. Antiseptics are chemicals that kill or prevent the growth of micro-organisms such as bacteria, viruses or fungi. The chemicals exert their antiseptic effect by slowly releasing iodine. Betadine may produce side effects, including wound irritation, rash or discomfort. In extreme reactions, altered thyroid function has been known along with decreased kidney function because of iodine absorption. Betadine ointment will be applied generously to small patches of David's burn wounds, particularly the buttocks and secured in place with a non-adherent dressing such as Telfa™, followed by adequate layers of gauze and crepe bandage to prevent the Betadine soaking through.

Biobrane cannot be applied if the burn is caused by hot fat or oil, or by flame, as the wound is most likely to be deeper than a superficial to partial-thickness wound. Cultural consideration and consent is also required because of the components within it. Biobrane is a biosynthetic wound dressing constructed of a silicone membrane bonded to a nylon mesh to which peptides from a porcine (pig) dermal collagen source have been bonded forming a flexible and conformable dressing. The majority of David's wounds will be dressed this way. Biobrane has a better chance of adhering to a wound if the wound bed is clean and free from contaminants, and therefore David's burns will be washed with chlorhexidine prior to application. The Biobrane will be overlapped onto normal skin by 0.5 cm to ensure that the wounds are covered fully and then secured in place using steri-strips, gauze and crepe bandage.

David's first wound check should take place 48 hours after application in order to check for adherence, collections of exudate underneath the Biobrane and for signs of infection. The next change of dressing will be dependent upon swab results and the clinical picture. If swab results remain negative for bacterial growth, the dressing should stay intact for 5 days.

6   Burns increase calorie usage. How is nutrition provided?

A   The basal metabolic rate may double after a major burn and can continue to increase up to 36 hours after the initial injury, causing a rise in energy consumption which lasts up to 12 days after the burn. The patient is at risk of muscle deterioration as a result of the protein and nitrogen losses that are used for energy production. Significant nitrogen losses can be identified by the presence of urea in the urine. Blood samples will be taken regularly to assess David's urea and electrolyte levels (U&Es).

David may require nasogastric intubation for additional feeding and calorie replacement. Unless contraindicated, enteral feeding is encouraged 24 hours after the burn in order to prevent further complications. At least 20 per cent of calories should be from protein. Carbohydrates provide a large number of calories for energy use. Fat intake also provides calories and meets the body's fatty acid requirements. A diet high in protein and carbohydrates with vitamin and mineral supplements is beneficial to the promotion of wound healing through the creation of essential amino acids. Close monitoring of the nutritional status of the patient must be ongoing, with support from a dietician.

7   What might be the long-term impact on David?

A   The depth of a burn wound and its healing potential are the most important determinants of the therapeutic management of the wound and potential scarring. David's burn injuries will have been assessed accurately using a multidisciplinary-team approach. His specific interests and needs stemming from his learning disability will have been assessed and met. He will have received appropriate pain relief, wound management and nutrition in order to optimize healing. Ultimately, though, the effects of receiving a large burn injury can last many years.

The impact of having a burn cannot be underestimated, and the required aftercare may be lengthy, addressing a number of issues (National Burn Care Review 2001). David's case is not a complex one, but he will go on to require continued physiotherapy support to maintain limb function and range of movement through passive exercises and stretching. This, along with occupational therapy support, will help to maintain new skin integrity and prevent skin contracture formation. Continuing wound care, pain management and nutritional support to maintain tissue viability and new skin integrity will also be required.

David's mother and his sister would have been traumatized initially by the accident, and, as with David, they will require continued emotional and psychological support from the burns clinical psychologist.

Answer to calculation exercise

3 x 55 (David's weight) = 165
165 x 11 (TBSA burn) = 1815

The medication needed would be 1815 ml over 24 hours.
Half (907 ml) will be given in the first 8 hours from the time of injury and the remainder over the following 16 hours.

> ## Key points
>
> - The treatment of burns is dependent upon objective assessment of the depth and extent of burned areas. Standard means of achieving this using TBSA, body surface area charts and internationally recognized classification of burns should be employed.
> - Fluid resuscitation, pain management and evidence-based selection of dressing technique are vital components of effective care.
> - When children have additional needs, such as David's learning disability, skilled nursing is required to adapt practice and to personalize care to their best advantage. Learning from parents and carers about children's specific needs and preferences remains important even in the presence of major injury.

REFERENCES

Bosworth Bousfield C (2002) *Burn Trauma: Management and Nursing Care, 2nd edn*. London: Whurr Publishers Ltd.

Forensicmed: Forensic Medicine for Medical Students (2015) *Assessment of Burns*. Available at: http://www.forensicmed.co.uk/wounds/burns/assessment-of-burns/ (accessed 24 January 2016).

Herndon D (2013) *Total Burn Care* (4th edn). St. Louis, MO: Saunders.

Kennedy R, Binns F (2014) Communicating and managing children and young people with autism and extensive burn injury. *Wounds* UK 10(3): 60–65. Available at: http://www.researchgate.net/publication/280712723_Managing_children_and_young_people_with_autism_and_burn_injuries (accessed 24 January 2016).

Lund CC, Browder NC (1944) The estimation of areas of burns. *Surgery, Gynecology & Obstetrics* 79: 352–358.

National Burn Care Review (2001) *Standards and Strategy for Burn Care*. London: NBCR.

National Institute for Health and Clinical Excellence (2010) *Clinical Guideline 112: Sedation for Diagnostic and Therapeutic Procedures in Children and Young People*. London: NICE.

Michael J (2008) *Healthcare For All: Report of the Independent Inquiry into Access to Healthcare for People with Learning Disabilities*. London: Aldridge Press.

Miller S, Aitken S (2003) *Personal Communication Passports: Guidelines for Good Practice*. Available at: http://bit.ly/Nh4lg1 (accessed 24 January 2016).

Monstrey S, Hoeksema H, Verbelen J, Pirayesh A, Blondeel P (2008) Assessment of burn depth and wound healing potential. *Burns* 34(6): 761–769 (DOI: 10.1016/j.burns.2008.01.009).

North West Children's Major Trauma Network (2015) *Clinical guidelines 2015*. Available at: http://nwchildrenstrauma.nhs.uk/_file/HrriLn9BBO_241096.pdf (accessed 24 January 2016).

Piira T, Sugiura T, Champion G, Donnelly N, Cole A (2005) The role of parental presence in the context of children's medical procedures: a systematic review. *Child: Care, Health and Development* 31(2): 233–243.

Pratt K, Baird G, Gringras P (2012) Ensuring successful admission to hospital for young people with learning difficulties, autism and challenging behaviour: a continuous quality improvement and change management programme. *Child: Care, Health & Development* 38(6): 789–797.

Royal Manchester Children's Hospital (2013) *Returning to School Following a Burn Injury a Guide for School Staff*. Manchester: RMCH. Available at: https://www.cmft.nhs.uk/media/313489/returning%20to%20school%20following%20a%20burn%20injury%20for%20schiool%20staff%2001.11.11.cm3730%20tig19%2007.pdf (accessed 24 January 2016).

Smith J, Atknson S (2012) Children who have difficulty in communicating, in V Lambert, T Long, D Kelleher (eds) *Communication Skills for Children's Nurses*. Maidenhead: McGraw-Hill, pp.152–170.

Tomlinson D, von Baeyer CL, Stinson JN, Sung L (2010) A Systematic review of faces scales for the self-report of pain intensity in children. *Pediatrics* 126(5): e1168-98 (DOI: 10.1542/peds.2010-1609).

Wong-Baker FACES Foundation (2015) *Wong-Baker FACES® Pain Rating Scale*. Oklahoma City (OK): Wong-Baker FACES Foundation. Available at: http://wongbakerfaces.org/ (accessed 24 January 2016).

Knife assault

Patric Devitt and Sue Rothwell

Case outline

Michael, aged 12 years, was walking home with his 13-year-old girlfriend, talking on the phone when two men attempted to snatch the phone from him. Initially, he resisted but released his phone when he felt a sharp stab to his right thigh. The men ran away immediately. With help, Michael managed to make his way to the paediatric emergency department and presented in the waiting room looking pale and with evident blood loss from his leg. His girlfriend was crying and screaming loudly for help, and the receptionist immediately called the nurse for assistance.

---

1 **What will be the nurse's first priority in this case?**

A As Michael has suffered a penetrating wound proximal to his knee he is commenced on the major trauma pathway. He is moved to the resuscitation room, and the major trauma team is summoned. Penetrating wounds to the thigh can be particularly serious because of the presence of so many nerves and blood vessels including the femoral, superior and inferior gluteal arteries, and the saphenous and femoral nerves. Every hospital that receives trauma patients will have a major trauma pathway that guides action in cases such as this. Details vary according to locally available services and practices, but the version applied here is typical.

2 **How is Michael's case assessed?**

A The nurse is responsible for the initial assessment of Michael using the approach outlined in advanced paediatric life support (APLS, Advanced Life Support Group 2015): A – airway, B – breathing, C – circulation. Michael clearly has a patent airway, his breathing is not visibly affected, but he is certainly losing blood from the wound. Rapid checks show that his observations are:

- pulse 108 bpm
- blood pressure 136/80
- respiratory rate 35
- O_2 saturation 96 per cent in air.

Additionally, capillary refill time is less than 2 seconds, and conscious level is 'A' using AVPU (Alert, Voice, Pain, Unresponsive; See Case 8). This indicates that his respiration, heart rate and blood pressure are all slightly elevated above the normal limits for his age.

3 **Why might you expect this?**

A This could be as a result of shock caused by Michael's injuries or as a physiological response to the body's release of adrenaline in preparation for fight or flight. Naturally, Michael has had a traumatic experience and is likely still to be agitated and demonstrating a stress response. It is particularly important to observe for changes in Michael's vital signs, recognizing that otherwise healthy young people can compensate for blood loss through raised heart rate, and classic signs of shock are late indicators.

INTERVENTION

Oxygen is administered at 10 L per minute by non-rebreathing facemask in the light of the evident blood loss and first recorded observations. Any seriously injured child (even if apparently well) requires intravenous access to be established as a matter of urgency in case of deterioration, to allow for fluid replacement or the need to administer drug therapy. Two relatively large intravenous cannulae are inserted into peripheral veins to ensure that venous access is readily available. In especially serious cases, when venous access may be impossible because of circulatory collapse, other options will be considered, including intra-osseous cannulation of a long bone. Intravenous fluid is administered in order to replace the loss from bleeding. As a result of the need for urgent treatment it is not possible to weigh Michael so an estimation must be made. APLS guidelines (Advanced Life Support Group 2015) for determining a child's are as follows.

0–12 months: weight (in kg) = (0.5 x age in months) + 4
1–5 years: weight (in kg) = (2 x age in years) + 8
6–12 years: weight (in kg) = (3 x age in years) + 7

Calculation exercise

Calculate Michael's approximate weight using the APLS formula. Michael requires 10 ml of replacement fluid per kg of body weight per 24 hours. How much replacement fluid should be given in the first 24 hours? How much fluid would be administered per hour?

The answer is given at the end of this case on p. 109.

Since there are no signs of shock, the maintenance fluid is sufficient. There is no need for an immediate bolus injection of fluid. If there were signs of circulatory compromise, uncontrolled bleeding must be considered and confirmed or excluded quickly. Surgeons who can deal with any of the injuries that are suspected should be called in immediately (if they are not already part of the trauma team) and the operating team alerted.

There is evidence that vigorous fluid administration is harmful in the presence of uncontrolled bleeding. The concern is that rapid normalization of blood pressure may disrupt early clot formation and dilute the clotting factors, leading to greater blood loss. Fluid resuscitation, therefore, depends on whether or not severe uncontrolled bleeding is suspected. For this reason it would be appropriate for children to be given aliquots of 10 ml/kg of crystalloid solution followed by rapid reassessment and subsequent 10 ml/kg as required. If 40 ml/kg of crystalloid has been administered to a child who remains unstable, blood should be used for further fluid replacement.

4 **Why should blood transfusion be employed rather than more crystalloid fluid?**

A Crystalloid and colloid solutions replace the diminished fluid volume in the circulation as well as replacing some of the electrolytes, but they do not carry oxygen. Only a blood transfusion can increase oxygen-carrying capacity quickly. Read more about resuscitation fluids in an article by Pryke (2004), together with more discussions of the topic on the same site.

INFECTION CONTROL MEASURES

At times of emergency it can be easy to forget about the risk of infection, but all bodily fluids, and particularly blood, should be considered as being potentially infectious. A number of simple, routine measures should be taken to prevent contamination: wearing protective clothing (non-sterile plastic apron, gloves, sometimes eye protection); effective hand-washing; cleaning of spilled blood with appropriate materials; and disposal of contaminated dressings, paper towels used for soaking up blood or cleaning the contaminated area. See the extensive guidance from Health Protection Scotland (2014); NHS Professionals (2013); and The Royal College of Nursing (2012). The videos provided by the National Patient Safety Agency (2011) on handwashing are particularly clear on how and when to wash the hands after contact with patients.

5 **What treatment will be provided?**

A Michael's care is coordinated initially by an emergency department consultant. However, assessment shows that there is no damage to either main blood vessels or major nerves so his care is transferred to the surgical team. To rule out any other soft tissue damage a magnetic resonance imaging scan is performed. Following this Michael is prepared for theatre to have the wound examined under general anaesthetic and sutured. Although it would be possible to undertake this under local anaesthetic, the Royal College of Anaesthetists (2012) suggests that employing general anaesthetic in children reduces anxiety and improves outcomes.

6 **What wound care is needed?**

A Since the wound will be sutured and dressed in theatre under general anaesthetic, no further wound care should be required until reviewed by community nursing staff some days later. These nurses will remove sutures or clips at the appropriate time and following skilful assessment of the wound and healing.

7   **What ethical issues are raised in relation to Michael and his injury?**

A   There are two ethical issues that you may be considering in relation to Michael's treatment and care following the assault. The first concerns whether or not he is able to consent to his own treatment (Wheeler 2006). Initially, the treatment that Michael requires is to prevent serious harm or death, and this cannot be delayed by the need to seek consent. However, once the condition is stabilized, efforts will be made to contact his parents to secure their oral consent to the proposed general anaesthetic and surgery. You would imagine that the nurse making this call would need to employ considerable skill in breaking the news while reassuring the parent that Michael is in no immediate danger. If the parents arrive in time, formal written consent will be obtained. If the parents cannot be contacted within a reasonable time, and assuming that Michael is in agreement, treatment would not be delayed to the detriment of his health.

The second area of concern is in relation to informing the police. In the UK, the Crime and Disorder Act 1998 permits health professionals to disclose confidential information to the police where they believe that such information could assist in preventing a crime or assisting an investigation. However, unlike the case with gunshot wounds, it is not a legal requirement (General Medical Council 2009). Obviously, if Michael wishes the police to be informed, the nurse will do so and provide contact details. However, if he does not, then it may still be that anonymized data will be given to the police for statistical purposes. Contact information in this case would only be provided if there was a convincing justification for doing so.

8   **What psychological care might Michael and his girlfriend require?**

A   In addition to the physical trauma he has suffered, Michael and, indeed, his girlfriend may feel psychologically affected by the events of the evening. Victim Support provides a specially tailored service for young people called 'You & co' (http://www.youandco.org.uk/) that helps young people to cope with the impact and effects of crime. It is not linked to the police and court system, and it maintains complete confidentiality. It is available both for victims and for witnesses of crimes. Michael and his girlfriend are provided with the contact details of the service.

9   **How soon would Michael go home?**

A   Since Michael has had surgery to explore and close his wound, he will require admission for at least a few hours, in this case, probably until the following morning. If he has managed to eat and drink, and can get around independently, he should be able to be discharged fairly soon afterwards. It would be advisable to ensure that he has a prescription for an analgesic and is aware of how and when to take this and any possible side effects. As he has had an anaesthetic and is a minor, he will not be allowed to go home unaccompanied, so he needs a responsible adult to collect him from the ward. His father picks him up in the morning.

10   **How would the safeguarding aspect of the case be pursued?**

A   A referral is made to the hospital's safeguarding team because of the type of injury sustained. A member of this team will check for any previous concerns about safeguarding issues linked to Michael, and will liaise with the school nurse in order that any existing concerns can be shared. A discharge letter is routinely sent to every patient's general practitioner on discharge to ensure that continuity of care is provided.

Answer to calculation exercise

36 + 7 = **43 kg**
(weight x 10 ml) 43 x 10 ml = 430 ml in 24 hours
430 ml ÷ 24 hours = **18 ml per hour**

Key points

- All hospitals have planned pathways in place for common scenarios: in this case, a major trauma pathway. These provide evidence-based structure and algorithms for decision-making. Familiarity with the most commonly used pathways would help you to understand what is happening in critical incidents and to play a useful supporting role.
- In some emergency situations estimations are needed (of approximate weight in this case). Application of such formulae prevents delays in intervention, ensuring effective fluid resuscitation.
- Protection of the public, other patients and staff is an important consideration in emergency department nursing, and there are legal requirements to report certain injuries. Although these requirements may seem confusing, senior staff will be able to explain the nuances of each case.

REFERENCES

Advanced Life Support Group (2015) *Advanced Paediatric Life Support*. Manchester: ALSG. Available at: http://www.alsg.org/uk/APLS (accessed 24 January 2016).

General Medical Council (2009) confidentiality: reporting gunshot and knife wounds. London: GMC. Available at: http://www.gmc-uk.org/Confidentiality__reporting_gunshot.pdf_55972947.pdf (accessed 10 February 2016).

Health Protection Scotland (2014) *National Infection Prevention and Control Manual*. Glasgow: HPS. Available at: http://www.documents.hps.scot.nhs.uk/hai/infection-control/ic-manual/ipcm-p-v2-3.pdf (accessed 24 January 2016).

National Patient Safety Agency (2011) *Five Moments*. London: NPSA. Available at: http://www.npsa.nhs.uk/cleanyourhands/resource-area/nhs-resources/education/five-moments/ (accessed 24 January 2016).

NHS Professionals (2013) *Standard Infection Prevention and Control Guidelines*. Watford: NHS Professionals. Available at: http://www.nhsprofessionals.nhs.uk/download/comms/cg1%20standard%20infection%20prevention%20and%20control%20guidelines%20v4%20march%202013.pdf (accessed 24 January 2016).

Pryke S. (2004) Advantages and disadvantages of colloid and crystalloid fluids. *Nursing Times* 100(10): 32. Available at: http://www.nursingtimes.net/clinical-subjects/cardiology/advantages-and-disadvantages-of-colloid-and-crystalloid-fluids/204444.fullarticle (accessed 24 January 2016).

Royal College of Anaesthetists (2012) *Raising the Standard: A Compendium of Audit Recipes.* London: RCOA. Available at: http://www.rcoa.ac.uk/ARB2012 (accessed 24 January 2016).

Royal College of Nursing (2012) Essential practice for infection prevention and control: Guidance for nursing staff. London: RCN. Available at: https://www2.rcn.org.uk/__data/assets/pdf_file/0008/427832/004166.pdf (accessed 24 January 2016).

Wheeler R. (2006) Gillick or Fraser? A plea for consistency over competence in children. *BMJ* 332: 807. Available at: http://www.bmj.com/content/332/7545/807.full (accessed 10 February 2016).

PART 5
Long-Term Conditions

CASE STUDY 14
Neonatal prematurity
Michaela Barnard and Louise Weaver-Lowe

Case outline

Jessica has just been transferred from the delivery unit to the neonatal intensive care unit (NICU). She was born prematurely 20 minutes ago at 28 weeks' gestation weighing 1.2 kg. She needed newborn life support (NLS) at birth, was intubated, and received her first dose of surfactant before transfer to the NICU. Jessica has been attached to the ventilator to support her breathing and her oxygen requirements are currently 40 per cent.

Jessica's mother remains on the delivery unit and her father is waiting in the parents' room to come and see Jessica as soon as her transfer to the unit is completed and Jessica is stabilized.

Jessica is being nursed in an incubator. She has an umbilical venous catheter (UVC) for intravenous hydration and an umbilical arterial catheter (UAC) for invasive blood pressure monitoring and blood gas sampling. As you begin to attach the monitoring equipment, you identify and document the physiological observations noting hypotension, with a mean arterial pressure (MAP) of 22 mmHg.

NEONATAL PREMATURITY

Babies born prematurely are normally considered viable at 24 weeks' gestation and resuscitation will be commenced at delivery (Figure 14.1). However, a neonatologist will attend some births below that gestation and undertake an assessment to confirm gestation, maturity and chance of survival. See Table 14.1 for categories of prematurity and low birthweight.

There are around 50,000 premature births in the UK each year. Preterm births account for 7 per cent of live births in the UK (Office for National Statistics [ONS] 2012). Initial resuscitation does not mean that all babies will survive past the neonatal period. The infant mortality rate in 2010 for preterm births in the UK was 24.3 per cent (ONS 2012). Long-term outcomes for babies who survive in the extremely preterm range are variable.

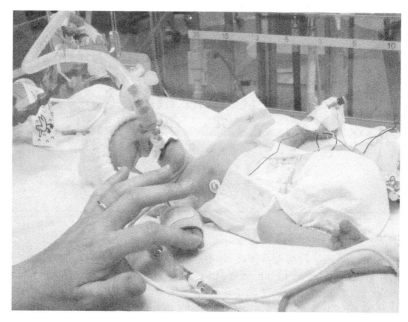

Figure 14.1 Neonate with ventilation

Table 14.1 Categories of prematurity and low birth weight

Gestation		Weight	
Preterm	<37 weeks	Low birth weight	<2500 g
Moderately preterm	35–37 weeks	Very low birth weight	<1500 g
Very preterm	29–34 weeks	Extremely low birth weight	<1000 g
Extremely preterm	24–29 weeks		

Normal physiological observations for a 28-week gestation baby such as Jessica are:

temperature: 36.8–37.2°C (axilla)
heart rate: 110-160 bpm
respiratory rate: 40-60 bpm
BP (MAP): 52 mmHg
SpO$_2$: 90–95 per cent.

1 **How would Jessica be assessed upon arrival to the NICU? Consider any frameworks of assessment that might be helpful. Show the priority given to the assessment approach.**

A Jessica will already have been assessed at delivery following the NLS guidelines (Resuscitation Council UK 2010). Any initial assessment after transfer of a sick, premature baby should follow an ABC approach, particularly as Jessica is intubated.

A – The endotracheal tube (ETT) size, length and position at the lips should be recorded.

B – Jessica should be observed for bilateral and equal chest movement. This can then be confirmed by auscultation. It is usual for a premature baby to synchronize with the ventilator breaths but also to have some spontaneous respiratory effort along-side this.

C – Jessica's colour and perfusion should be assessed. Jessica may have some resid-ual peripheral cyanosis after delivery, but this should resolve within a few hours of birth. Jessica should look centrally pink with pink lips. Perfusion can be assessed quickly and non-invasively by measuring capillary refill time (CRT). This should be measured by applying sufficient pressure to blanch the skin on the central area of the chest with the index finger for 5 seconds. The finger should then be removed and seconds timed until the blanching skin returns to the original colour. A blanching time of two to three seconds suggests satisfactory perfusion, whereas more than three seconds requires further assessment and investigation. It should be noted that CRT is a subjective test and it should not be used as an indicator of circulatory status in isolation.

Jessica would then need assessment of her temperature, firstly an axilla measure-ment, then skin temperature monitoring can be placed for continuous recording. Full monitoring of respiratory rate, heart rate (including QRS waveform), SpO_2, non-invasive blood pressure (NIBP) and invasive blood pressure should be undertaken. Jessica's skin should be observed for any marks. The nappy should be observed for urine output and/or meconium.

2 **Think about the early administration of surfactant and consider why surfactant has been administered immediately. How does natural surfactant act in the small airways and why is the lack of surfactant problematic for premature babies?**

A Surfactant production occurs naturally, and secretion in the fetal lung begins between 24 and 28 weeks' gestation but is not complete until 35 weeks' gestation. Surfactant reduces the surface tension in the alveoli enabling a maximum surface for gaseous exchange (Figure 14.2).

Surfactant deficient lung disease (SDLD) is a lead cause of mortality in premature infants. Surfactant deficiency leads to alveolar collapse and poor gaseous exchange (Sweet et al. 2013). In Jessica's case, due to her birth weight and gestation, she is at risk of SDLD. She has already had one dose of surfactant in the delivery room either for prophylaxis or rescue during resuscitation. One or two doses of surfactant are nor-mally sufficient to achieve the required result. A baby must be intubated for surfactant to be administered. The baby needs to be in a midline neutral position prior to admin-istration. A catheter is then passed down the ETT and the small volume of surfactant is injected as a single bolus. The therapeutic response to surfactant can be immediate, requiring rapid alterations in ventilation and oxygen requirements as gaseous exchange improves. Endotracheal suctioning should be avoided for four hours after administra-tion of surfactant.

CUROSURF® (poractant alpha), is administered as a single endotracheal bolus and is provided at a concentration of 80 mg/ml in two sizes of vials, either a 1.5 ml or a 3 ml vial. The dose of surfactant should be prescribed as in Table 14.2.

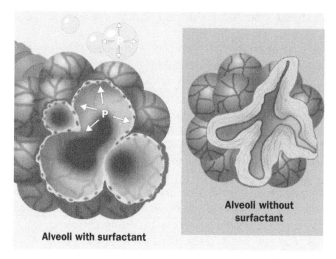

Figure 14.2 Neonatal lungs with and without surfactant

Table 14.2 Birth weight and dose of CUROSURF

Birth weight	600—1200 g	1201–2400 g	2401–3600 g
Dose	120 mg	240 mg	360 mg

Source: Paediatric Formulary Committee 2014.

Calculation exercise

Jessica has been prescribed surfactant. Before administration, you need to check that the dose is correct. What dose should Jessica be prescribed? What volume should be delivered by endotracheal bolus? Should the dose be repeated, if so, when?
The answer is given at the end of this case on p. 121.

---

3   **Thermoregulation in premature neonates is a priority. Discuss why thermoregulation is important and what nursing interventions would be needed to maintain Jessica's temperature.**

A   There are four mechanisms of heat loss that will put Jessica at risk of hypothermia. These are conduction, convection, evaporation and radiation. Conduction would occur when heat is lost if in contact with a solid surface, for example, a cold towel on delivery. Convection is when heat is lost to air currents, such as a draught or open incubator doors. Evaporation occurs when heat is lost through evaporation of fluid, such as through the skin or breathing. Radiation is when heat is lost from the skin to a colder surrounding surface such as the incubator walls.

Neonatal skin is a significant factor in thermoregulation as it is the main organ responsible for heat loss. The skin of a premature neonate is underdeveloped, thin and prone to damage. It provides inadequate insulation and babies will lose heat very quickly.

At delivery, Jessica should have been placed into a plastic bag, in preference to drying and wrapping (Leadford et al. 2013). This intervention provides better temperature control in the first 24 hours together with a pre-heated incubator. Humidity can be introduced into the incubator for infants of less than 28 weeks' gestation. This will encourage the process of keratinization of the skin, where a hardened layer of protein is formed in the skin cells, preventing heat and water loss. Jessica will need continuous temperature monitoring.

4 **Think about the causes of hypotension in a neonate. What risks to Jessica's condition could be caused by hypotension? How could Jessica's hypotension be monitored and managed?**

A The causes of low blood pressure in premature infants include hypovolaemia, sepsis, intra-ventricular haemorrhage, infection and cardiac problems. Prolonged hypotension will compromise the perfusion of vital organs, such as the brain and kidneys, potentially resulting in long-term damage to these organs. Babies with hypotension may also present with pallor, poor perfusion and tachycardia.

Initially, Jessica's hypotension should be monitored closely. The MAP in neonatal blood pressure is the most significant reading that guides clinical decision-making. Invasive (UAC or arterial line) and non-invasive blood pressure measurements should correlate closely. In invasive monitoring, calibration and placement of the arterial transducer should be checked initially and after any position changes to ensure accuracy of blood pressure recording. The arterial trace on the monitor should have a strong, bounding wave. The expected blood pressure for preterm babies is represented in Table 14.3.

Inotropic drugs would be administered to manage Jessica's hypotension. Inotropes facilitate the delivery of oxygenated blood to vital organs by stabilizing and maintaining blood pressure. They increase cardiac contractility without affecting the heart rate. In premature neonates, careful adjustment of the dose and monitoring is needed. Dopamine and dobutamine are common inotropes administered by continuous intravenous infusion.

A number of medications used in neonatal care are unlicensed for neonates and therefore are produced in adult concentrations. Calculations of these medications are complex and neonatal nurses undergo further numeracy training and assessment to achieve the level of competency required.

5 **Jessica has umbilical arterial and venous catheters. Think about their function and situation on and inside the body. What nursing care is needed to maintain the safety of these catheters?**

A There are three blood vessels in the umbilical cord: one vein and two arteries. The UAC is inserted by a doctor into one of umbilical arteries and passed to a point high at the level of the diaphragm or low below the level of the renal arteries (Figure 14.3). An x-ray

Table 14.3 Expected blood pressure by gestation

Gestation (weeks)	23–27	28–32	33–36	37 onwards
BP (MAP) mmHg	22–42	52	56	63

BP, blood pressure; MAP, mean arterial pressure.

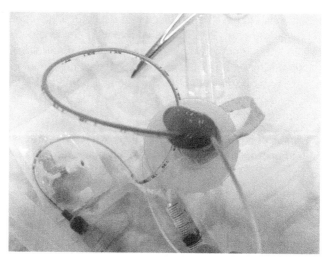

Figure 14.3 Cannulation of umbilical vessels

is taken to confirm correct placement. The UVC is inserted into the umbilical vein and its final position is measured and confirmed by x-ray. The UVC can be used for administration of fluids and medication, or for central venous pressure monitoring.

Close observation of the UAC and UVC are needed to ensure patency and to reduce the risks of infection, phlebitis or compromised perfusion to the limbs. Both catheter sites should be cared for using ANTT (Aseptic Non Touch Technique [http://antt.org/ANTT_Site/home.html]: an internationally accepted approach to prevent health care infections), and the entry sites should be observed hourly for bleeding, oozing, redness and inflammation. Key indicators of problems are pressure increases on the infusion pump, any difficulty sampling the UAC, or a poor trace on the blood pressure wave form. When a UAC is in place, particular observation must be made of the lower limbs and buttocks for changes in colour, warmth or blanching (due to obstruction of the arterial supply). Medical staff would need to be informed immediately of changes to limb perfusion and removal of the UAC would be considered.

6 **Having a baby on a neonatal unit is a significantly stressful and emotional experience for parents. Consider Jessica's admission from her parents' perspective and generate a list of potential concerns that they may have.**

A Premature labour and consequent delivery of a premature baby is often an unexpected experience. Babies like Jessica are unwell at delivery, requiring immediate care and intervention, resulting in separation from their parents. Parents often do not get to see their baby properly before they are taken to the neonatal unit. These events are outside of the expected normality previously imagined by the parents and can cause considerable emotional strain. Feelings of shock, guilt and disempowerment are common. The neonatal environment is often intimidating for parents especially when they see their small baby connected to and surrounded by large pieces of noisy equipment.

Read this extract from a real-life account in which Jenny, mother of Charlee born at 28 weeks' gestation, describes her feelings:

I felt helpless, comforted, overwhelmed, amazed, scared, hopeful, shocked and reassured, usually at least 3 of them at the same time, but most definitely all of them at some point in a 24 hour period. It's without doubt the most daunting place I've ever been, but at the same time is strangely comforting. It's a total roller-coaster of an experience, where you're trying to focus on the smallest of positives without being consumed by the negatives.

Parental bonding is promoted by touching and holding the baby. Being able to hold their baby at an early stage is key to forming an emotional attachment (Klaus and Kennell 1976). Admission to a neonatal unit and the need for intensive care is an immediate barrier to effective parental bonding.

Family-centred care should be a core philosophy of any neonatal unit and nurse, where the parents' and family's needs are considered a key aspect of caring for the baby. Parents should feel empowered in their parental role by nurses who communicate effectively and teach them how to undertake some of the practical caregiving needs for their baby. Development of a secure therapeutic relationship, initiated by the nurse, is a crucial factor in facilitating parental roles (Roberts et al. 2015). Some parents may need further psychological care and referral to deal with the emotions and stress arising from this difficult event in their lives.

Extra resource

Watch this You Tube clip to develop your understanding of a parent's perspective of life on a NICU (https://www.youtube.com/watch?v=ROqYOlZjeJO).

Jessica is now 2 years old and has come to the outpatients department for her 2-year follow-up appointment with the consultant. Jessica's parents have some concerns about her eyesight and her cognitive and motor development.

Some children who have been born prematurely are left with ongoing health and developmental problems such as cerebral palsy. Approximately 1,800 children are diagnosed with cerebral palsy every year and premature birth increases the likelihood of this condition (Hemming et al. 2008). Children such as Jessica are followed up in a clinic to review their development, to develop a plan of care for health problems and to be referred to other health professionals as required. Jessica will have had some developmental assessments already from her health visitor in the community, and these will feed into the review.

7   **Think about the potential problems that Jessica might have at this age. What areas of development do you think the consultant might want to assess?**

A   Initially, the consultant will listen to the concerns that Jessica's parents have. This will also allow the doctor to observe Jessica's behaviour and any interactions. Assessment will be made to identify any functional disability and specifically if there is cerebral palsy. Developmental tests will be applied and results will categorize if Jessica has normal development, mild, moderate or severe delay. Some children may also present with hydrocephalus and history of seizures. Jessica will be assessed for gross motor ability, sensory and communications ability or disability. Somatic function will be assessed, identifying ongoing problems with respiration, renal function, gastrointestinal tract and establishing growth patterns.

8   **Jessica wears glasses and her parents are concerned about her eyesight. What is a causative factor of ongoing eye problems following premature birth?**

A   Some children who were born prematurely will have visual impairment. This can range from blindness to mild impairment. Some children may have severe impairment as a result of cerebral haemorrhage, hypoxic ischaemic injury or retinopathy of prematurity.

Retinopathy of prematurity (ROP) is more likely in low birth weight babies and those babies born before 32 weeks' gestation. Retinopathy of prematurity occurs when immature blood vessels of the retina start to grow abnormally. This abnormal growth is triggered by a number of factors including the amount of oxygen treatment that the baby receives and the baby's general clinical condition. These blood vessels are weak, can bleed, and scar the retina, sometimes causing detachment in very severe cases. Retinopathy of prematurity is classified in stages, with stage 1 being mild and stage 5 being complete detachment. Premature infants have regular eye examinations by the ophthalmologist and treatment can be planned for those infants with a severe enough disease to jeopardize the baby's sight. Treatment is normally laser therapy. The severity of ROP can be limited in the neonatal period by the strict regulation of oxygen. All neonatal units have guidelines for lower and upper limits of SpO_2 according to gestation, in order to limit the damage excessive oxygen can do to developing retinal blood vessels.

Jessica will have received regular eye examinations on the neonatal unit and any extent of ROP should be documented and discussed with her parents. In addition, premature birth can inflict a number of challenges on Jessica's developing ocular system in addition to ROP. The ophthalmologist would be able to advice on visual impairment and long-term outcome.

The future for children like Jessica can be full of uncertainty. Her parents will have hopes and dreams for her future. However, they are likely to experience significant anxiety regarding her ability to function and develop as an independent person and their ability to support her through childhood and into adulthood.

Answer to calculation exercise

Jessica weighs 1.2 kg, or 1200 g, so the correct dose is 120 mg, and a single 1.5 ml vial is required. Since at most two doses of surfactant are required, and Jessica has already had one dose in the delivery room, then no further doses will be expected after this one.

Key points

- Although assessment algorithms for neonates are similar to those for other children, anatomical and physiological differences demand additional skills of observation and interpretation in the nurse.
- Thermoregulation is a vital concern in neonatal nursing, especially so for premature babies, while respiratory support, often with administration of surfactant, is a further specific need.
- The ability to rescue babies born prematurely can come at a cost, with physical and sensory consequences. Continuing follow-up of the children is needed to ensure the optimum outcome.

REFERENCES

Hemming K, Colver A, Hutton JL, Kurinczuk J, Pharoah POD (2008) The influence of gestational age on severity of impairment in spastic cerebral palsy. *Journal of Pediatrics* 153(2): 203–208.

Klaus MH, Kennell JH (1976) *Parent-Infant Bonding*. St Louis, MO: Mosby.

Leadford AE, Warren JB, Manasyan A, et al. (2013) Plastic bags for prevention of hypothermia in preterm and low birth weight infants. *Pediatrics* 132(1): 128–134.

Office for National Statistics (2012) *Gestation-Specific Infant Mortality in England and Wales, 2010*. London: ONS.

Paediatric Formulary Committee (2014) *British National Formulary for Children*. London: BMJ Publishing Group, Pharmaceutical Press and RCPCH Publications.

Resuscitation Council UK (2010) *Newborn Life Support*. London: Resuscitation Council. Available at: https://www.resus.org.uk/pages/nls.pdf (accessed 24 January 2016).

Robert J, Fenton G, Barnard M (2015) Developing effective therapeutic relationships with children, young people and their families. *Nursing Children and Young People* 27(4): 30–35.

Sweet DG, Carnielli V, Greisen G, et al. (2013) European consensus guidelines on the management of neonatal respiratory distress syndrome in preterm infants – 2013 update. *Neonatology* 103: 353–368.

A child with newly diagnosed type 1 diabetes mellitus who is in transition from primary to secondary school

Tony Long and Jude Campbell

Case outline

Sam, aged 10, has been admitted to the paediatric ward from the accident and emergency department (A&E). He is accompanied by his father. He had attended the general practice surgery earlier that day with symptoms of tiredness, polyuria, polydipsia and weight loss. His blood glucose level was found to be abnormally high with measurable ketonuria. A diagnosis of type 1 diabetes mellitus (T1DM) was made. On admission he is generally well, not significantly dehydrated and able to drink without problems. Other than hay fever and a tendency to catch coughs and colds easily, Sam has no other medical history. He enjoys energetic team sports, and despite problems with performance and stamina recently, he has also become a successful competitive runner in a local athletics club. He is accompanied by his father, who seems to be more anxious than Sam about the diagnosis.

The diagnosis has been confirmed quickly from the history and through routine and specific blood tests (blood glucose, HbA1c (glycosylated haemoglobin), glutamic acid decarboxylase (GAD) and islet cell antibodies, and blood gasses. Random blood glucose was found to be 15 mmol/l, while blood ketones were found to be 2.0 mmol/l.

---

1 **What is type 1 diabetes mellitus?**

A Type 1 diabetes mellitus results from the effects of lack of natural insulin production by the beta cells of the islets of Langerhans in the pancreas. This prevents the metabolism of sugar and carbohydrates, and also disrupts fat and protein metabolism. The cause of diabetes is unknown, although genetic inheritance seems to be implicated in a minority of cases, and environmental factors may also play a role. Type 1 diabetes mellitus occurs in children and young people, with peak incidence between 10 and 14 years (Department of Health 2007a). This long-term condition is common in the UK, and the incidence is increasing steadily. In 2011 the incidence in children 0–14 years of age was 24.5 per 100,000 – the world's fifth highest rate (Diabetes-UK 2012).

2   **What do you think are the main issues to be addressed before Sam can go home? (Consider treatment, routine monitoring, knowledge and preparation for occasional problems).**

A   The main aim of treatment for T1DM is to re-establish glucose metabolism and stabilize blood glucose levels through administration of insulin and dietary control. Effective management and control of diabetes reduces or delays the impact of common long-term complications, especially microvascular problems (Department of Health 2007a; International Society for Pediatric and Adolescent Diabetes 2011; Royal College of Paediatrics and Child Health 2009). It also promotes more immediate benefits of improved school attendance and attainment, and support for engagement in sport and other healthy activities.

As you read the next few sections, try to keep in mind the perspective of children like Sam: the enormity and permanence of the changes in his life, and the deep desire just to be a normal child.

INSULIN INJECTIONS/INSULIN PUMP THERAPY

Most children in Sam's situation are treated best by a regime of intensive insulin therapy. This might be by multiple injections or continuous subcutaneous infusion (insulin pump). At diagnosis the total daily dose is calculated at 0.5 units per kg body weight. The notion of multiple injections for the rest of his life might be daunting for Sam. This is recognized by organizations supporting children with diabetes and age-appropriate literature is available to help patients and parents to understand and cope with this (see Diabetes UK [https://www.diabetes.org.uk/], Diabetes Ireland [https://www.diabetes.ie/]).

The family will have to know about and to be able to manage several issues:

- understand the function of insulin and its effects under varying circumstances
- work out insulin doses and know when to augment this based on carbohydrates consumed and on blood glucose levels
- load an insulin pen and dial the dose
- administer the injection
- site rotation
- dispose of sharps safely
- how to store insulin and equipment.

BLOOD GLUCOSE AND BLOOD KETONE MONITORING

The dose of insulin is adjusted according to blood glucose levels. Self-monitoring of blood glucose should be undertaken four times daily: before breakfast, lunch and evening meal, and finally before bed. At first, an additional test during the early hours (2–4 am) is helpful in eliciting the pattern of blood glucose and the response to insulin. National guidelines (National Institute for Health and Clinical Excellence [NICE] 2015) provide target blood glucose levels:

- 4–7 mmol/L before meals
- 5–9 mmol/L two hours after a meal
- 4–7 mmol/L on waking.

Stability is an important factor, so the personal target levels for individual children may vary in order to avoid severe or frequent hypoglycaemia.

3   What are ketones?

A   Ketones (or ketone bodies) are produced when fat is metabolized in the absence of sufficient insulin to move glucose from the blood into the cells. In normal metabolism, glucose, insulin and ketones are part of a balanced system of making energy available to the body (for example, during exercise), but this balance is upset in hyperglycaemia. This might happen if the planned dose of insulin is insufficient or if an insulin pump blocks or fails. Ketones are acidic and toxic – leading to diabetic ketoacidosis (DKA) which, if left untreated, leads to confusion, loss of consciousness and coma (Figure 15.1). On the ward, blood ketones will always be checked whenever blood glucose rises higher than 13.9 mmol/L. At home, Sam or his parents will test for blood ketones if he becomes ill, if the blood glucose rises above the level set for him on the ward (usually 14mmol/L) or if he shows any signs of DKA.

   Sam and his parents will need to learn how to test for blood glucose and ketones and to show understanding of the impact of blood glucose levels together with the implication of finding more than 0.6 mmol/L ketones on testing. A home testing kit for blood glucose and ketones will be provided.

4   What is hypoglycaemia, and how is it managed?

A   Hypoglycaemia (blood glucose below 4.0 mmol/L) results gradually from a mismatch between food consumed, insulin dose and recent exercise, and is characterized by unpleasant, embarrassing and potentially dangerous symptoms (Clarke et al. 2009). Some potential episodes of hypoglycaemia can be anticipated such as during exercise,

Diabetic ketoacidosis (DKA)
Persistent thirst
Polyuria
Nausea or vomiting
Blurred eyesight
Flushed or dry skin
Difficulty in breathing
Tiredness
Confusion

Figure 15.1 Symptoms of diabetic ketoacidosis

Table 15.1 Signs of hypoglycaemia

Early signs	Later signs
Cold sweating	Slurred speech
Shaking or trembling	Inability to concentrate
Hunger	Irritability
Rapid pulse (maybe palpitations)	Confusion and irrational behaviour
Anxiety	Unconsciousness
Tingling sensation in the lips	Coma (perhaps with convulsions)

and action can be taken to reduce the risk of them occurring. However, many are unpredictable so Sam, his parents, his friends and his school teachers need to be able to recognize the early signs of impending hypoglycaemia and, especially, the signs of more severe problems (Table 15.1).

RESPONDING TO MILD OR MODERATE HYPOGLYCAEMIA

On recognizing the onset of hypoglycaemia, Sam should take some refined carbohydrate the amount will depend on the age and weight of the child, in Sam's case approximately 15 g of carbohydrate would be a sensible initial recommendation: glucose tablets or full-sugar drinks act quickly and produce a rise in blood sugar. Other sources (milk, chocolate and biscuits, for example), take longer to release sugar because of the fat content and would therefore not be recommended. Sam should have this worked out in his plan. The blood glucose will be tested again after 15 minutes. If the blood glucose is no better, then more glucose should be taken. If it is improving, then a snack or the next meal (complex carbohydrate) may be taken to prevent recurrence. If Sam is using an insulin pump then only refined carbohydrate needs to be given. There is no need to give any complex carbohydrate for follow-up treatment.

TREATMENT OF SEVERE HYPOGLYCAEMIA – GLUCAGON

If the blood glucose worsens and signs of severe hypoglycaemia appear such as unconsciousness or a compromised airway, then more urgent treatment is needed as Sam will not be able to take anything orally. He needs to be positioned in the semi-prone (recovery) position, and glucagon will be injected intramuscularly.

5 **What is glucagon?**

A The hormone glucagon is also produced in the islets of Langerhans of the pancreas, but in the alpha cells (rather than the site of insulin production – the beta cells). Normally, it works in harmony with insulin to maintain the blood glucose level after a high protein meal. Insulin causes the amino acids to be used for protein synthesis (muscle growth and repair), while glucagon acts to promote uptake of the amino acids by the liver for conversion into energy through a process of gluconeogenesis. In this way, the body's needs for both energy and protein synthesis are met, and the blood glucose remains stable.

In diabetes, however, the lack of insulin to counterbalance glucagon can lead to a dangerous rise in blood sugar some time after a high-protein meal. Glucagon raises the blood sugar as expected, but this is compounded by the availability of additional amino acids for gluconeogenesis. This mechanism can be used to good effect, though, if the blood sugar falls drastically such that a hypoglycaemic episode occurs, rapid restoration of blood sugar levels can be achieved by injecting glucagon. On recovery, vomiting is common (Clarke et al. 2009), and recurrent hypoglycaemia could occur. Close monitoring of the blood glucose is needed.

Usually, when severe hypoglycaemia has occurred, the family or the school will have called for paramedics to attend. The paramedics will administer the glucagon (if it has not already been given), and then wait with the child until consciousness is regained and the child can take oral food and drink. If parents are still unsure that recovery is progressing, then the child is admitted to hospital. All families are instructed to inform the diabetes team if glucagon has been used for treatment of hypoglycaemia, and such incidences are followed up by the team.

6 **What is the routine for management of hyperglycaemia?**

A Even the best routine of insulin injection cannot replace the natural mechanism, so episodes of hyperglycaemia will occur sometimes. Blood glucose levels appearing high can be caused by a variety of factors – inaccurate calculation of insulin dose against carbohydrate intake, poor injection technique or lipohypertrophy, and other reasons. However, concern should be felt if signs other than high blood glucose appear – polyuria, polydipsia, fatigue, or, more importantly, ketonaemia. Additional rapid-acting insulin should be injected as decided in the plan based on the individual insulin sensitivity factor (ISF).

As children and young people grow, develop and move through puberty their bodies will require significant increases in insulin dosages. The occurrence of frequent hyperglycaemia is often an indication that insulin dosages need to be reviewed. If blood ketones are recordable and greater than 0.6mmol/L then extra instructions and a more aggressive management plan needs to be commenced. Blood ketones are produced when the blood glucose renal threshold is breached (approximately 13.9 mmol/L).

SICK DAY MANAGEMENT

Although children with well-controlled diabetes should not experience any more illness than other children (Brink et al. 2009), illness still occurs. Illness (particularly infection) affects diabetic control.

7 **Suppose that you were going to explain this to Sam. See how much you have understood and remembered yourself, and write a brief explanation suitable for Sam.**

A You might have produced something like this. Fighting infection uses more energy, so liver and muscle stores are accessed. More insulin is required to move this additional glucose into the cells. Without sufficient insulin, fat is metabolized instead, leading to the production of ketones and eventually DKA. However, low blood glucose is possible, too, particularly if vomiting and diarrhoea are experienced. Just as with anyone else who feels ill, Sam might not feel able to tolerate eating.

It is important for Sam to understand and follow **sick day rules**.

Rules if the blood glucose is low during a sick day

(1) If the blood glucose is low but not less than 5 mmol/L, then Sam must take his usual insulin dose and substitute sugary drinks if carbohydrate as a meal or snack cannot be faced.

(2) If the blood glucose is below 4 mmol/L, then only background insulin should be given, and 10–20 g of carbohydrate as a sugary drink should be taken (amount depending on body weight, but this is what Sam should take).

(3) If this low blood glucose persists, then the next dose of background insulin should be halved.

(4) Blood glucose levels should be checked every one to two hours.

Rules for high blood glucose during illness

(1) *Never stop taking normal insulin.* Even if Sam is eating less than normal, this baseline insulin is needed for normal metabolism and to use glucose produced from stores. Ketones will be removed only if insulin has been administered.

(2) *Do more blood tests.* Checking the blood glucose every one to three hours might be necessary until ketones have been removed. It is vital for Sam to understand what is happening with his blood glucose profile.

(3) *Check for ketones in the blood if blood glucose rises above 14 mmol/L.*

(4) *Take plenty of water, sugar-free or no-added-sugar or diet drinks to help with removal of ketones.*

(5) *Eat carbohydrate foods.* Despite being ill, indeed because of this, carbohydrates are still needed for energy. Sugar-containing drinks can be used to replace meals or snacks when necessary. Hydration also must be maintained with regular sugar-free drinks such as water. Give extra fast-acting insulin to remove ketones. The dose will be documented in Sam's individual plan and is likely to be calculated by giving the normal ISF correction dose of insulin with an added 10–20 per cent dependent on the level of ketones present. One to two hourly blood glucose testing should be performed with strict rules for Sam and his family to access medical advice if hyperglycaemia and ketonaemia is not improving within 2–4 hours.

Sam and his parents should never be reluctant to consult the diabetes team if they are unsure or concerned. Vomiting or extremes of blood glucose should prompt them to seek professional help (Brink et al. 2009). Additional medication might be needed (as with anyone else), such as antibiotics (Diabetes Ireland 2014).

DIET AND EXERCISE

8 **What sort of carbohydrate is contained in different foods?**

A Different foods contain different types of carbohydrates:

- *starchy carbohydrate* – potatoes, rice, pasta, noodles, bread, cereals, couscous, lentils and beans
- *fructose* – fruit and fruit juice
- *lactose* – milk, yoghurt, ice cream, and custard
- *sucrose* – table sugar.

Some carbohydrates are fast-acting. They are digested quickly and cause a rapid rise in blood glucose. Some carbohydrates are digested more slowly, prompting a more gradual rise in blood glucose. In diabetes it is best to include slow-acting carbohydrates to prevent fluctuations in blood glucose (see Table 15.2 – those carbohydrates in italics are particularly slow-acting).

It is imperative to be able to count the number of carbohydrates in a meal or snack in order to select food wisely and to calculate the amount of insulin required. Children, of course, tend to be fond of snacks, so wise choices need to be made about these. Read the snack list in Table 15.3 and see if there are any surprising items. Most multiple daily insulin regimens require the individual with diabetes to cut down on snacks between meals to prevent the need for insulin injections to be given. Advice from dieticians suggests that only one snack per day of less than 10 g of

Table 15.2 Slow-acting and fast-acting carbohydrates

Slow-acting carbohydrates	*Fast-acting carbohydrates*
Breakfast cereals: Weetabix, *Porridge, Shreddies*	Sugary drinks (including fruit juice)
Breads: *wholegrain, granary*	Sweets
Pasta and noodles	Table sugar
Rice *basmati*	Glucose tablets
Beans	Lucozade/energy drinks
Milk	
Fruit	

Carbohydrates in italic are particularly slow-acting.

Table 15.3 Snack List (10 g carbohydrate or less)

Food item	Carbohydrate (g)
Low sugar jelly pot	2
Squeezy yoghurt (40 g)	6
Small pot (50 g) fromage frais	6
1 bread stick	4
1 cream cracker	5
1 rice cake	5
2 poppadums	6
1 bag Wotsits	10
1 bag Skips	9
1 small plain biscuit	10
50 g peanuts	5
25 g mixed nuts and raisins	9
6 strawberries	6
Small apple	10
Satsuma	5
100 ml fruit juice	10
200 ml milk	10
Options/highlights hot chocolate drink	5

carbohydrate is advisable. However, some younger children will require more than this to provide enough daily nutrition.

CARBOHYDRATE-COUNTING EXERCISES

Normal meals also need to be carbohydrate-counted in the same way. Use the extensive list at the following web link offered by Diabetes UK (2011) to see how food that you eat measures up (http://www.diabetes.org.uk/upload/How%20we%20help/catalogue/carb-reference-list-0511.pdf). Then try the exercises below, checking yourself against the Diabetes UK list.

9   **Which items in these meals contain carbohydrate, and how many grams of carbohydrate?**

(1) Two rashers of bacon, a fried egg, two tablespoons of beans, and two thick slices of toast.
(2) Two tablespoons of cornflakes with 200 ml milk.
(3) Pasta bowl with chicken pieces, followed by an apple and a handful of grapes.

Calculation exercise

Sam's blood glucose, insulin and food chart states that he should have the following.

- Carbohydrate ratio = 1 unit novorapid/humalog for each 10 g carbohydrate (CHO) at breakfast, lunch and tea.
- Correction = 1 unit novorapid/humalog will reduce blood glucose by 3 mmol/L.
- Target blood glucose is 6 mmol/L.

At breakfast, Sam's blood glucose was 12 mmol/l. He ate two slices of toast (30 g), and a glass of milk (10 g). Calculate how much insulin he should take.

For lunch, he had an egg sandwich with two slices of bread (30 g), a yoghurt (20 g), an apple (15 g) and crisps (15 g). His blood glucose was 9 mmol/L. How much insulin should he take?

For supper, Sam had two slices of thin crust pizza (35 g) and two scoops of vanilla ice cream (15 g). His blood glucose was 6 mmol/L. How much insulin is needed?

The answer is given at the end of this case on p. 134.

---

10   **Should diabetic children engage in exercise?**

A   Children and young people with diabetes should feel no limitation on the ability to excel in their chosen sports, and all should experience the same opportunities and access as others in the population for exercise, leisure and health pursuits (Robertson et al. 2009). The body's response to intense or prolonged exercise differs between people with diabetes and people who do not have diabetes. However, the response can be predictable for different types, intensity and longevity of exercise, so sensible planning beforehand will do much to prevent dramatic swings in blood glucose. Regular exercise, with associated adjustment of metabolic systems, is less problematic than irregular and varied exercise.

For most general school sports, and for a boy of Sam's age, a small snack of about 10-15 g carbohydrate – a sports bar or a piece of fruit – taken before exercise provides extra carbohydrate for use during the exercise and allows replenishing of glycogen stores afterwards (preventing a rebound period of hypoglycaemia). Insulin may also need to be reduced before exercise (perhaps by 20–25 per cent) since additional blood glucose will be used up as fuel for the exercise. Without reducing the insulin, hypoglycaemia could result. Detailed advice and individual exercise-planning schedules can be tailor-made for children and young people taking part in frequent competitive sports.

11   **The management of physiological aspects of Sam's care is complicated and extensive. This is only one side of Sam's needs, though. What should be done regarding psychological and emotional well-being?**

A   You probably noted that Sam's father was understandably anxious, and the same education package that is applied to Sam is also relevant for his parents. Understanding the condition and the means to minimize long-term problems is important in addressing the father's concerns. Parental adjustment to the diagnosis, and working through their grief for the loss of their child's normal healthy life can be serious problems. Involvement of a clinical psychologist when the diagnosis is discussed with parents is now standard and an accepted part of treatment for patients and their family. Access to counselling should be routine, while specialist professional expertise in mental health should be available to the clinical team (Department of Health 2007b; International Society for Pediatric and Adolescent Diabetes 2011). Annual psychological screening should be routine with timely signposting to child and adolescent mental health services if problems are identified (NICE 2015).

Even if not of immediate interest to Sam, there will be other psychological and emotional challenges for him in the future. The never-ending routine of dietary management, blood monitoring, and insulin administration unavoidably has an impact on leisure, relationships and activity, restricting some ambitions and conflicting with teenage desires for independence and feelings of rebellion. NHS Diabetes and Diabetes UK (2010: p. 6) refer to 'the demands of the condition and the demands of life, and the interaction between the two' influencing the level of need for psychological or emotional support, and note that intensification of emotional need is likely to undermine everyday self-management. Clearly, times of major transition (such as moving to secondary school) prompt greater emotional need.

> Since Sam will be going to secondary school in a few months' time, it is important to identify the changes that will occur and to prepare for the additional challenges that these will bring.

12 **What do you think the problems might be, and how would you prepare Sam, his parents, and his teachers to cope with them?**

A Sam has two tasks to accomplish. First, he has to learn about his condition and how to manage this to remain healthy both immediately and in the long term. Then he has to maintain this in a new school environment in which his routines will become disrupted and in which he will not want to appear to be different to his peers.
You might have thought about the following.

- Technical skills of insulin administration, and blood glucose and ketone testing.
- Maintaining a healthy diet while also carbohydrate-counting and managing the demands of exercise and sport.
- Management of episodes of hypoglycaemia and hyperglycaemia.
- Adjusting to growth spurts and different daily routines (being more or less active at different times).
- Maintaining a place in his much-expanded peer group.
- Oh yes – and studying, too.

Moving to secondary school involves a change to more self-disciplined approaches, reliance on students themselves to identify their own needs and to seek solutions to their problems. In some ways, this might be seen as paralleling the gradual (though more accelerated) development to self-management of diabetes, so perhaps the move towards independence will be helpful. However, in a larger school and with an ethos of self-management, there is a danger that acute warning signs of hypoglycaemia or hyperglycaemia may not be identified by others. There is often a mismatch in responsibilities between parents and children in regard to who is responsible for different aspects of diabetes management. This mismatch often becomes more noticeable during transition to secondary school. It is imperative that children and their parents continue to communicate daily in regard to blood glucose testing results and insulin dosages if blood glucose control is to remain optimized during transition.

Although there may have been an awareness of Sam's particular dietary needs in those serving food at primary school, it is more unlikely to be the case in secondary school, so accurate carbohydrate-counting will be even more important for Sam. His meal times may vary from day to day, and sometimes the school day can be longer at secondary school. He will have days with sports sessions for which he will need to adjust his insulin doses. As a result of these challenges, most children and young people with diabetes take a packed lunch from home so that carbohydrate counting can be done at home and an insulin dose can be attached to this. Effectively, at lunchtime Sam will need to do a blood glucose test and calculate his correction insulin to add to the dose already suggested for his carbohydrate in his lunch.

Guidance on the management of medicines in schools, together with associated proformas and advice on constructing local plans and strategies was provided by the Department of Education and Skills and the Department of Health in 2005, and there are many resources for children, parents and teachers on the Diabetes UK website. National and regional diabetes care plans are available and form part of a tripartite agreement between home, school and diabetes teams.

13　**Overnight trips are a common part of the curriculum to encourage personal growth in pupils. Like all of his peers, Sam will not want to be different or to seem in any way weaker or less able than others. Think about the additional issues that he will have to consider to be well while exploiting the opportunities of joining in the trip and its associated activities.**

A　You probably thought of some of these.

- The type, frequency, and carbohydrate content of food supplied on the trip.
- Availability of a suitable environment in which to do blood testing and injecting.
- The type and frequency of activities.
- The likelihood of insulin-adjustment training of accompanying staff.
- Emergency contact numbers.
- Holiday or trip medical insurance.
- Insurance for all of the equipment (insulin pump, testing materials).
- Restrictions on certain activities (for example, some roller-coasters).

With planning, these can all be overcome and Sam ought to be able to join in and enjoy himself as much as everyone else. The emphasis needs to be placed on being prepared so as to allow activity rather than to focus on restrictions and non-participation.

This information should be passed to the parents and Sam so that the family can be prepared for the particular areas in which Sam may struggle in coming months as he starts at his new school.

Answers to calculation exercise

Breakfast: Sam takes 40 g CHO, so he needs 4 units (4 x 10 g). He is already 6 mmol/L over his target, so he needs 2 additional units in correction (2 units per each additional 3 mmol/L). Total = 6 units.

Lunch: he has 80 g CHO. 8 x 10 g = 8 units of insulin. He is already 3 mmol/L over his target, so he needs an additional 1 unit of insulin. Total = 9 units.

Supper: the blood glucose is on target, so no correction dose is needed. 50 g CHO (5 x 10 g) requires 5 units of insulin.

Key points

- From the earliest opportunity children are encouraged to understand and take responsibility for their own diabetic control. This is important since self-management will be a lifelong task, and since the building of sound knowledge and positive attitude is essential to the self-discipline of diabetic control.
- Carbohydrate counting, blood glucose testing and calculation of insulin requirement are central to maintaining health and diabetic control, so nurses must be able to teach, check, advise or correct children's knowledge or practices in these areas.
- Sick day management rules are a central aspect of control, particularly during the school years. School trips and normal sporting activities should remain an integral part of life.

REFERENCES

Brink S, Laffel L, Likitmaskul S, et al. (2009) Sick day management in children and adolescents with diabetes. (ISPAD Clinical practice Consensus Guidelines 2009 Compendium.) *Pediatric Diabetes* 10 (Suppl. 12): 146–153 (DOI: 10.1111/j.1399-5448.2009.00581.x)/

Clarke W, Jones T, Rewers A, Dunger D, Klingensmith GJ (2009) Assessment and management of hypoglycaemia in children and adolescents with diabetes. (ISPAD Clinical practice Consensus Guidelines 2009 Compendium.) *Pediatric Diabetes* 9: 165–174. (DOI: 10.1111/j.1399-5448.2009.00583.x).

Department of Health (2007a) *Making Every Young Person with Diabetes Matter*. London: Department of Health. Available at: https://www.diabetes.org.uk/documents/reports/makingeveryyoungpersonmatter.pdf (accessed 25 January 2016).

Department of Health (2007b) You're Welcome Quality Criteria. *Making Health Services Young People Friendly*. London: Department of Health. Available at: http://webarchive.nationalarchives.

gov.uk/20130401151715/https://www.education.gov.uk/publications/eorderingdown-load/275246.pdf (accessed 25 January 2016).

Department for Education and Skills and Department of Health (2005) *Managing Medicines in Schools and Early Years Settings*. London: DfES. Available at: https://www.gov.uk/government/uploads/system/uploads/attachment_data/file/196479/Managing_Medicines.pdf (accessed 25 January 2016).

Diabetes Ireland (2014). *Managing your Child's Diabetes*. Available at: https://www.diabetes.ie/living-with-diabetes/child-diabetes/managing-childs-diabetes/ (accessed 10 February 2016).

Diabetes UK (2011). *Carbohydrate Reference List*. London: Diabetes UK. Available at: http://www.diabetes.org.uk/upload/How%20we%20help/catalogue/carb-reference-list-0511.pdf (accessed 24 January 2016).

Diabetes UK (2012) *List of Countries by Incidence of Type 1 Diabetes Ages 0 to 14*. Available at: http://www.diabetes.org.uk/About_us/News_Landing_Page/UK-has-worlds-5th-highest-rate-of-Type-1-diabetes-in-children/List-of-countries-by-incidence-of-Type-1-diabetes-ages-0-to-14/ (accessed 25 January 2016).

International Society for Pediatric and Adolescent Diabetes (2011) *Global 2011 IDF/ISPAD Guideline for Diabetes in Childhood and Adolescence*. Berlin: ISPAD. Available at: https://www.ispad.org/?page=IDFISPAD2011 (accessed 25 January 2016).

NHS Diabetes and Diabetes UK (2010) E*motional and Psychological Support and Care in Diabetes*. Available at: https://www.diabetes.org.uk/About_us/What-we-say/Improving-diabetes-healthcare/Emotional-and-Psychological-Support-and-Care-in-Diabetes/ (accessed 25 January 2016).

National Institute for Health and Clinical Excellence (2015) *Diabetes Type 1 & Type 2 in Children and Young People: Diagnosis & Management*. NG 18. London: NICE. Available at: http://www.nice.org.uk/guidance/ng18/resources/diabetes-type-1-and-type-2-in-children-and-young-people-diagnosis-and-management-1837278149317 (accessed 25 January 2016).

Robertson K, Adolfssen P, Riddell M, Scheiner G, Hanas R (2009) Exercise in children and adolescents with diabetes. (ISPAD Clinical practice Consensus Guidelines 2009 Compendium). *Pediatric Diabetes* 10 (Suppl. 12): 154–168 (DOI: 10.1111/j.1399-5448.2009.00567.x).

Royal College of Paediatrics and Child Health (2009) *Growing Up with Diabetes: Children and Young People with Diabetes in England*. London: RCPCH. Available at: http://www.rcpch.ac.uk/system/files/protected/news/FINAL_CYP_Diabetes_Survey_Report_(3)[1].pdf (accessed 25 January 2016).

A baby with short gut, referred to tertiary services following presentation with failure to thrive

Tony Long and Jane Roberts

Case outline

Eithne is 3 months old and breastfed. She was born at normal gestation but with gastroschisis: a congenital defect that allows abdominal contents to protrude through a defect in the abdominal wall. Routine sonography had revealed the presence of the defect during pregnancy, so the birth was conducted at a regional centre. Surgery was undertaken to remove a necrotic section of the ileum, leaving 50 cm of healthy ileum. The abdominal wall was repaired, and after four weeks Eithne was taken home.

After a further eight weeks, on examination in a clinic, her weight had fallen back to her birth weight of 3.6 kg, she was passing frequent loose stools, she was lethargic and clearly failing to thrive. Her mother was clearly anxious for the baby and feeling guilty that she had not sought help earlier.

1   Why might this have happened to Eithne? Reviewing what the normal bowel is like in a healthy infant is a good place to start. Ensure that you are familiar with the three parts of the small intestine. For an unusual perspective on how children might understand this see the explanation of 'Worms and washing machines: how the intestine works' by the Short Gut Syndrome Families' Support Group (Jackson 2015). With 50 cm remaining of the ileum, how much is likely to have been lost?

(a) 300 cm
(b) 10 cm
(c) 150 cm

A   The small bowel of a term infant is about 300–350 cm long. The duodenum may be about 7.5 cm long, and the jejunum and ileum make up the remaining part with a ratio of 2:3. The right answer is (c) (about 150 cm). In this case 75 per cent of the ileum has been lost.

2 **How do the functions of the duodenum, jejunum and ileum differ?**

(a) **The duodenum and jejunum absorb nutrients and water.**

(b) **The duodenum breaks food down whereas the jejunum and ileum absorb nutrients and water.**

(c) **They all do the same thing.**

A Although the boundaries of the sections of small bowel are not finely defined visually, the functions of the stomach and duodenum are to start the process of digestion breaking food down and adding secretions such as saliva and bile. The jejunum and ileum work to reabsorb the huge volume of water that is added to the intestine and to capture nutrients, vitamins and electrolytes through specially adapted sites. The right answer is (b).

3 **How much of the fluid that enters the intestinal tract is reabsorbed into the blood-stream by the jejunum and ileum together?**

(a) **20%**

(b) **50%**

(c) **80%**

A The right answer is (c). By the time matter is passed through into the caecum, approximately 80 per cent of the fluids that are ingested or secreted by the body itself in digestive processes have been reabsorbed. Missing sections of ileum have a significant impact on this function, further exacerbated by failure to absorb bile salts that pass into the large bowel causing it to lose more water, causing the dangerous loss of fluid in Eithne's case. The ileum's reduced ability to reabsorb water while also failing to absorb vital nutrients including vitamin B_{12}, carbohydrate, protein and electrolytes leads to diarrhoea and failure to thrive.

Immediate treatment

As Eithne presents as a seriously ill baby who may require surgery to lengthen the gut and remove any non-viable tissue, the major concern is to make her fit for surgery through rehydration, rebalancing of electrolytes and supply of nutrients.

PARENTERAL NUTRITION

Restoring Eithne's nutritional state is achieved by parenteral nutrition through a central venous access catheter. Careful monitoring of electrolyte levels, trace elements and the pH of the blood is vital. Blood tests will be conducted daily (full blood count, urea and electrolytes [kidney function], and liver function tests). Regular monitoring by nurses of pulse, blood pressure and respirations is important to detect early signs of problems with fluid balance.

Infection and parenteral nutrition

The feeding solution is made up of fats and high percentage glucose which are dense in calories and which have been lost through malabsorption. With such a nutrient-rich content, parenteral nutrition poses a serious infection risk to the baby. Strict guidelines provided by the Association for Safe Aseptic Practice (2014) will be followed. Monitoring of the temperature will be maintained in order to recognize indications of infection.

Breastfeeding

Although health professionals should make every effort to encourage and support breastfeeding of babies even when unwell, in this case breastfeeding will have to be ceased since oral breast milk will not be absorbed. However, with support from a breastfeeding consultant or advisor, Eithne's mother may be able to maintain lactation until such time as oral feeding can be resumed. The mother's need for psychological and practical support with this vital aspect of childcare should not be underestimated or ignored.

Indications of progress

Eithne will be weighed twice weekly to assess progress. Parenteral nutrition is prescribed according to body weight. Regular weighing is required to ensure that the correct fluid and nutritional requirements are provided. Large weight gains and losses can be due to fluid retention or losses, and these need to be taken into consideration when parenteral nutrition is given.

Corrective surgery

After three weeks Eithne is sufficiently recovered to undergo surgery. The operation involves removing a further 20 cm of necrotic ileum near to the jejunum and lengthening of the remaining ileum.

A number of procedures are adopted to achieve this, often by splitting the remaining dilated ileum lengthways, suturing the halves into tubes and joining these tubes together end to end (the Bianchi or autologous procedure). A common alternative is the STEP (serial transverse enteroplasty) procedure. A simple explanation of this is provided for parents by the National Institute for Health and Care Excellence (2007).

> **Extra resource**
>
> You can watch the STEP procedure being undertaken in the You Tube video from Boston Children's Hospital (2012, https://www.youtube.com/watch?v=Zjl7AjiyXwQ).

4 **What do you think will need to be included in the care and treatment plan after the initial recovery from the surgery and healing of the wound? Think about monitoring homeostasis, re-establishing feeding, ongoing practical and psychological support, and return to normal development.**

(A) MONITORING HOMEOSTASIS

Although the surgery is designed to improve absorption dramatically, this improvement is gradual. It remains vital to record accurate fluid balance measurements. Eithne's mother and family will be included in this once they have received instruction in the important aspects of this.

ENTERAL FEEDING

At first, parenteral nutrition will be continued. Hopefully, Eithne's mother will already have helped with this and can continue to do so post-operatively. Intestinal feeding is reintroduced gradually once intestinal function has returned (Amin et al. 2013). Oral feeding is promoted and encouraged. If additional support is required in the short term, a nasogastric tube may be used, but the emphasis will be on returning as quickly as possible to oral feeding. Returning to normal feeding may take a long time and requires patience and perseverance. Loose stools may continue for many months or even years, so nursing support for the children and families is necessary until stools are thicker and more controllable. If the mother has been breastfeeding, then the aim is to return to this, although additional support may be required from a breastfeeding counsellor. Expressed breast milk will be used at first until the baby is able to suck well, with gradual return to normal breastfeeding (Rudolph et al. 2010). If this seems to be difficult in practice, reflect on what is achieved in far more difficult circumstances (Emergency Nutrition Network 2004).

PRACTICAL AND PSYCHOLOGICAL SUPPORT

Eithne will remain a more difficult baby to manage than usual. A prolonged period of recovery and gradual development of normal gastrointestinal function means that her mother will require ongoing support. This starts in the hospital from surgical nurses and specialist gastroenterology nurses, but must continue seamlessly once Eithne goes home. Outreach undertaken by the specialist nurse and early liaison with community children's nurses are central to this. Additional support may be found from other parents whose children have had similar problems and surgery, and this can be accessed in the UK through the Short Bowel Survivor and Friends forum (http://www.shortbowelsurvivor.co.uk/) and dedicated Facebook site.

HEALTH AND DEVELOPMENT

Eithne's continued development will be monitored by her health visitor, who will also provide advice and support about nutrition and childcare as Eithne progresses to reach total intestinal autonomy. A dietician will play an important role in ensuring optimal nutritional status. Qualified play specialists will have an important role in adapting toys and games to promote Eithne's physical and psychological growth. This is all the more important in view of the constraints of the illness and long periods of unusual lifestyle. There is always an expectation of a normal childhood, however, especially if successfully weaned off parenteral nutrition.

Home parenteral nutrition is undertaken routinely now nationally and internationally. Training families to become competent as experts in their own child's care is a significant task in terms of staff time, although the ability to care for the child at home is clearly a motivating factor. Once Eithne is established with parenteral nutrition at home continued support is required by specialist nursing and nutrition staff from the hospital as well as routine support from community nurses. Infection during the use of parenteral nutrition remains a particular risk. Extensive guidance is available from the National Clinical Guideline Centre (UK) (2012). Undertaking parenteral nutrition at home can itself represent a stressor for parents, so ready access to advice, problem-solving and reassurance will be vital for Eithne's parents for some time to come during the long period of extended recovery.

Extra resource

Finish this case by reading Danielle's Story at the Short Bowel Survivor and Friends website (2015, http://www.shortbowelsurvivor.co.uk/#/dannielles-story/4553506472).

Key points

- Knowledge of the anatomy and functions of different parts of the intestine is essential to understanding the reasons for presenting signs and post-operative problems observed in a baby with short gut syndrome.

- Nursing care to ensure restoration of fitness for surgery through parenteral nutrition is a central pillar of treatment, and management of the associated risk of serious infection is crucial.
- Much psychological and practical support is needed by families who take a baby home after surgery or for home parenteral feeding. Specialist and community children's nurses will be a valued resource for families during the extended recovery period.

REFERENCES

Amin SC, Pappas C, Iyengar H, Maheshwari A (2013) Short bowel syndrome in the NICU. *Clinical Perinatology* 40(1): 53–68 (DOI: 10.1016/j.clp.2012.12.003).

Association for Safe Aseptic Practice (2014) *Aseptic Non Touch Technique – Core Guidelines*. Available at: http://antt.org/ANTT_Site/core_guidelines.html (accessed 25 January 2016).

Boston Children's Hospital (2012). *STEP Procedure Video from Boston Children's Hospital*. Available at: https://www.youtube.com/watch?v=Zjl7AjiyXwQ (accessed 25 January 2016).

Emergency Nutrition Network (2004) *Infant Feeding in Emergencies*. Oxford: ENN. Available at: http://www.unhcr.org/45f6c9e02.pdf (accessed 25 January 2016).

Jackson (2015) *Worms and Washing Machines: How the Intestine Works*. Taylorsville, UT: Short Gut Syndrome Families' Support Group. Available at: http://www.shortgutsupport.com/articles/how_the_intestine_works.php (accessed 25 January 2016).

National Clinical Guideline Centre (UK) (2012) *Infection: Prevention and Control of Healthcare-Associated Infections in Primary and Community Care: Partial Update of NICE Clinical Guideline 2*. London: Royal College of Physicians. Available at: http://www.ncbi.nlm.nih.gov/books/NBK115271/ (accessed 10 February 2016).

National Institute for Health and Care Excellence (2007) *Surgical Lengthening of the Bowel for Children with Short Bowel Syndrome*. London: NICE. Available at: http://www.nice.org.uk/guidance/ipg232/resources/surgical-lengthening-of-the-bowel-for-children-with-short-bowel-syndrome-307799965 (accessed 10 February 2016).

Rudolph JA, Squires R (2010) Current concepts in the medical management of pediatric intestinal failure. *Current Opinion in Organ Transplantation* 15(3): 324–329 (DOI: 10.1097/MOT.0b013e32833948be).

Short Bowel Survivor and Friends (2015). *Dannielle's Story*. Available at: http://www.shortbowelsurvivor.co.uk/#/dannielles-story/4553506472 (accessed 25 January 2016).

A teenager with chronic renal disease awaiting transfer from paediatric services to adult services

Tony Long and Trish Smith

Case outline

Tariq is a 16½-year-old boy who was diagnosed with juvenile nephronophthisis at the age of 8 years. He initially presented with polyuria, polydipsia, poor growth and renal impairment. Over time his kidney function gradually deteriorated resulting in established renal failure (ERF). Tariq has required overnight peritoneal dialysis for the past 18 months.

---

1   **See how much you remember about normal kidney function, and list three essential ways in which the kidneys help to maintain homeostasis.**

A   You will have remembered immediately that the kidneys remove water-soluble waste products of metabolism from the body. They also excrete drugs and their residual compounds. Constancy in composition of the blood is essential to health, and the kidneys play the major role in regulating body water content. Together the lungs and the kidneys regulate the acidity of the blood. The blood pressure is regulated partly by the kidney's varying absorption or excretion of sodium chloride. Finally, through excretion of hormones, the kidneys help to keep bones and teeth healthy, as well as contributing to blood cell production. There are other functions, too: kidneys are important organs.

FILTRATION AND REABSORPTION IN THE KIDNEY

Each kidney is made up of about a million filtering units called nephrons. The nephron includes a filter, called the glomerulus, and a tubule. The nephrons work through a two-step process. The glomerulus lets fluid and waste products pass through it; however, it prevents blood cells and large molecules, mostly proteins, from passing. The filtered fluid then passes through the tubule, which sends needed minerals back to the blood-stream and removes wastes.

JUVENILE NEPHRONOPHTHISIS (MEDULLARY CYSTIC DISEASE)

This is a rare inherited kidney disorder characterized by formation of cysts inside the kidney, kidney fibrosis and tubular atrophy, which leads to progressive kidney failure and ERF requiring dialysis and transplantation by adolescence. This autosomal recessive form accounts for 10–20 per cent of ERF in children, occurring equally in males and females (MacRae Dell and Avner 2003) (see the explanation of inheritance in Case 20). It is worth spending some time reviewing the Infokid site (www.infokid.org.uk) to see how kidney disease is explained to families.

PERITONEAL DIALYSIS

Dialysis removes toxins and regulates the amount of water in the blood. Peritoneal dialysis uses the peritoneum, which is the lining of the abdomen. A dialysate fluid is introduced into the abdomen, where it sits for a few hours while the peritoneum filters the blood. The used fluid is drained out of the body. This can take place in several cycles overnight using an automated machine such as the one in Figure 17.1. The composition of the dialysate can be altered to remove more or less fluid. Dialysis therapy provides only about 5–10 per cent of normal kidney function. Although this is enough to keep someone alive it brings limitations to normal health, and the treatment itself can have side effects.

2 **Consider some of the physical aspects of renal failure that Tariq has to contend with.**

A Tariq may be experiencing some of the following problems.

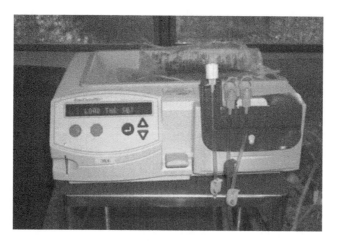

Figure 17.1 The Baxter Homechoice dialysis machine

ANAEMIA

Normal healthy kidneys produce the hormone erythropoietin, which stimulates the bone marrow to produce new red blood cells. In renal failure this hormone production is reduced so Tariq needs to have a subcutaneous injection up to three times each week. He will require ongoing treatment to keep his haemoglobin level above 110 g/l, which will then limit symptoms of anaemia.

LETHARGY

Renal failure results in the build-up of urea in the blood, and inadequate dialysis can result in lethargy. Tariq, although undergoing peritoneal dialysis, may still have less energy than his peer group, which can limit the activities in which he is able to participate.

Activity

In order to better understand the patient's problems, think for a few minutes about what having less energy means for someone of Tariq's age and the importance of peer group activity and identity.

DIALYSIS THERAPY

Tariq has to have his dialysis treatment for ten hours overnight, six nights per week. He or his parents have to set up the dialysis machine in the evening with all the bags of fluid that he will require overnight to enable him to connect up as he goes to bed. This takes about 30 minutes and needs to be done in a clean environment with particular attention to handwashing. Although the treatment takes place overnight while Tariq is sleeping, the machine may alarm during the night, disrupting his sleep or that of his parents. Tariq needs to ensure that he takes active care of his peritoneal dialysis catheter with attention particularly to the prevention of infection. It may well seem that there is never a day off and never a break from the treatment.

SHORT STATURE

Renal failure may well cause Tariq to be considerably shorter than his peer group, which will exert both physical and psychological impacts on him. Daily injections of synthetic growth hormone can help to treat short stature in some children; however, even with treatment children will often remain shorter than their peers.

Note that the problems are piling up here. As well as lacking the energy to keep up with his active peer group, Tariq is also likely to be physically smaller and weaker than them.

BONE DISEASE

Regulating the amount of calcium in the body is a complex problem. Too much calcium can lead to calcification of soft tissues (including blood vessels), whereas too little causes osteopenia (low bone mass) and can lead to cardiac arrhythmias. Three hormones are essential to normal calcium control: parathyroid hormone – which raises the amount of calcium in the blood by releasing it from bones; vitamin D or calcitriol (strictly, it is not really a vitamin but a hormone) – which aids absorption of dietary calcium; and calcitonin – which reduces circulating calcium and promotes its excretion through the kidneys. In renal disease, the production of calcitriol is reduced, leading to reduced intestinal absorption of calcium.

Phosphorus, a mineral that is essential in the bones, is intimately linked to calcium metabolism. Its level in the blood is usually regulated by excretion through the kidneys. Since this mechanism is compromised in chronic renal disease, the phosphates have to be bound up in other compounds (phosphate binders) to prevent absorption of dietary phosphorous (and leading to excretion through the bowel).

Tariq will need to take medication every day to keep his bones strong and healthy. Alfacalcidol (active Vitamin D) and phosphate binders are usually required.

DIETARY AND FLUID RESTRICTIONS

Close monitoring will be required of the amount of fluid drunk each day, as peritoneal dialysis will remove only a certain amount of extra fluid from the body. As progressive renal failure causes urine output to reduce over time, Tariq will need to limit the amount of fluid that he drinks. He may be able to have only 800–1000 ml of fluid a day. He will also have to limit the amount of potassium, sodium, protein and phosphate in his diet. The restrictive nature of this diet may be surprising.

3   **Look at the list of potassium containing foods in Table 17.1 and consider how difficult it is to avoid these foods as a young person. Would the alternative options be welcoming to you? How well does this fit with normal healthy eating messages?**

At 16½, Tariq is approaching a period of major transition in both life and health services. Adapting to dialysis treatment is difficult for any child and family. Managing this through adolescence and into young adulthood is another challenge to be faced. Moreover, as time goes by, renal function is increasingly compromised, complications occur more frequently and transplantation will be essential eventually. As a result of other health problems, there is no close relative who could be considered as a living donor for Tariq.

Table 17.1 Alternative low-potassium foods

	Potassium-rich foods to avoid	Lower potassium alternative
Drinks	Pure fruit juice Ribena Coffee Milky drinks	Weak tea Squash Fizzy drinks Water
Fruit	Apricots Bananas Grapes Oranges Dried fruit	Apples Pears Tinned fruit – without juice
Vegetables	Baked beans Tomatoes Tomato puree Mushrooms Brussels sprouts	Carrots Cauliflower Green beans Peas Sweetcorn
Cereal foods	Chocolate cake Chocolate biscuits Fruitcake Bran cereal Tinned spaghetti Instant noodle pot snacks	Wafers Plain and cream biscuits Jam-filled sponge Jam doughnuts Cream crackers Crumpets Bread sticks
Sweets and snacks	Chocolate Toffee Fudge Potato crisps Nuts Liquorice	Boiled sweets Mints Marshmallows Wheat-based snacks Corn-based snacks Wheat Crunchies, Wotsits, Skips, Popcorn
Miscellaneous	Chocolate spread Tomato ketchup Soup Yeast extract Salt substitutes	Jam Honey Marmalade Jelly

4 **Try to put yourself in Tariq's place and consider some of the issues that he and his family will be facing at this time of his life or in the foreseeable future. Think about what life would be like for most other teenagers at this time, and particularly the desire for independence. What effect might there be on his aspirations, and what might change in his health services?**

A Tariq will be pondering many questions not only about his treatment but also concerning the changes that he will have to face as he approaches his 18th birthday: transition from paediatric care to adult care; from full-time education to further education or the workforce; and dependence to independence. All of these transitions are difficult but they are made more complex by a chronic illness requiring daily medical treatment (Royal College of Nursing 2013a).

PAEDIATRIC TO ADULT CARE

Children and young people who have spent years receiving care within a paediatric centre find the thought of moving to new adult services daunting. They are anxious that no one will know them or understand what they have been through, and that other patients in adult care will be so much older. Parents are often more anxious than the young person and need help to ensure that this transition is managed well. This reflects a normal tension that is heightened for young people with chronic renal disease between a desire for independence and the unavoidable dependence on parents and other adults.

Many young people travel long distances to receive their renal care in a specialist tertiary children's service (there are only 12 of these centres in the UK). Transitioning to adult services provides an opportunity to receive specialist care nearer to home. The dialysis nursing and medical team will ensure that there are joint meetings between paediatric and adult professionals along with the child and family prior to the young person transferring completely to adult care. Specialist paediatric renal nurses and adult renal community nursing teams work closely to effect this smooth transition. The Royal College of Nursing (2013b) provides guidance and a clinical pathway for young people's transition to adult services.

FULL-TIME EDUCATION TO WORKFORCE

Completing full-time secondary education is a landmark for young people. Many choose to seek employment at this stage, although this can be more difficult because of their ongoing health needs. Others elect to continue to university (which also poses challenges). Whichever choice is made, young people in ERF need support to pursue their aspirations while maintaining their dialysis treatment.

DEPENDENCE TO INDEPENDENCE

Living with a chronic illness is difficult for the young person and their family. Ongoing support and assistance from their family is crucial for young people to manage their medical treatment yet most young people strive to live an independent lifestyle. Parents often struggle to allow the young person the freedom that they need while still providing essential help with their treatment. Parents may be more risk-averse than their offspring with ERF.

> **Extra resource**
>
> Explore the British Kidney Patient Association (www.britishkidney-pa.co.uk) and the Infokid (www.infokid.org.uk) websites to see the sort of support that is available.

ONGOING TREATMENT AND PLANNING FOR THE FUTURE

The Department of Health (2004) sets standards of care for people like Tariq. The importance of care planning and the provision of information to facilitate shared decision-making are emphasized: 'All children, young people and adults with chronic kidney disease are to have access to information that enables them with their carers to make informed decisions and encourages partnership in decision-making, with an agreed care plan that supports them in managing their condition to achieve the best possible quality of life' (Standard one, Department of Health 2004). Tariq will be aware that he will require peritoneal dialysis until he receives a successful kidney transplant. He will also know that the longer he waits for a transplant, the more likely it is that he will develop problems on dialysis as a result of infection or other complications of long-term therapy. This may well result in having to change to hospital-based haemodialysis three times each week: another restriction on his life.

Planning for the future is always difficult when managing a chronic illness. Even making plans to go on holiday with dialysis, although possible, is often too complex and stressful for a family to embark upon. This can have an effect on siblings and the family as a whole. The young person on dialysis often feels responsible for other family members also being restricted.

Waiting for a kidney transplant is difficult, too. Many young people are fortunate to have a family member who is able to provide them with a living donor organ, where everything can be planned well ahead of time, often preventing the need for dialysis at all. Tariq is in the unfortunate position where his family is unable to pursue this course of treatment due to their own health needs. Therefore, he has to wait for a suitable kidney donor to become available; which may take up to ten years in some cases.

ONGOING NURSING CARE

Specialist nurses are key members of the multiprofessional team and often have the closest relationships with the young person and their family. They provide ongoing care and education not only in hospital but also within the home environment, linking into schools, workplaces and voluntary organizations related to the young person's activities. They are well-placed to ensure that the young person and their family have the right practical guidance, emotional support and psychological help to ease their transition.

Key points

- Progressive renal disease with multiple associated problems and the restrictions of dialysis places psychological, social and physical pressures on the individual and their family.
- Transition from child-focused to adult services can be anxiety-provoking, particularly since this will be unfolding at the same time as other major life changes such as leaving school. Any deterioration in renal function is likely to be highlighted against this backdrop.
- Specialist nurses and patient groups play a vital role in supporting families during the trying years of haemodialysis and the anxious wait for a transplant opportunity.

REFERENCES

Department of Health (2004) The National Service Framework for Renal Services – Part One: Dialysis and Transplantation. London: DH. Available at: https://www.gov.uk/government/uploads/system/uploads/attachment_data/file/199001/National_Service_Framework_for_Renal_Services_Part_One_-_Dialysis_and_Transplantation.pdf (accessed 10 Feburary 2016).

MacRae Dell K, Avner ED (2003) Renal manifestations of systemic disorder. In RJ Postlethwaite, NJA Webb (eds) *Clinical Paediatric Nephrology (3rd edn)*. Oxford University Press.

Royal College of Nursing (2013a) *Adolescent Transition Care: RCN Guidance for Nursing Staff*. London: RCN. Available at: https://www2.rcn.org.uk/__data/assets/pdf_file/0011/78617/004510.pdf (accessed 10 February 2016).

Royal College of Nursing (2013b) *Lost in Transition: Moving Young People between Child and Adult Health Services*. London: RCN. Available at: https://www2.rcn.org.uk/__data/assets/pdf_file/0010/157879/003227_WEB.pdf (accessed 10 Feburary 2016).

PART 6
Emotional and Mental Health

Autism spectrum disorder

Janice Grant and Frances Binns

Case outline

Zack, aged 4, lives with his parents Joanne and Paul and his 8-year-old sister. Zack was born by forceps extraction after a prolonged and difficult labour. As a baby he was described as being 'good' as he was not very demanding and achieved most of his developmental milestones within the expected times for the first 18 months. Zack's speech was slow to develop, although this did not give immediate cause for concern as his older sister, Harmony, appeared to understand him and his needs. His social development was also apparently normal for the first 18 months. However, Joanne began to notice that Zack appeared to become upset when his routine was changed, and he liked to play with the same toys over and over.

At around the age of 2½ years, Zack's language skills appeared to be regressing, and although he spoke, his speech was high-pitched and comprised of repetitive words and phrases from his favourite Thomas the Tank Engine DVD. Joanne realized that Zack was using strange mannerisms repeatedly, rarely made direct eye contact and preferred to play alone with very specific toys. At the age of 3 Zack was diagnosed as being on the autism spectrum.

Currently Zack has very strong food preferences. He dislikes any changes in routine and becomes aggressive when anything in his routine is disturbed. He is particularly sensitive to loud noises, and his favourite activity is to put his toy cars in specific size and colour order. He also likes to watch the same Thomas the Tank Engine cartoon repeatedly, becoming engrossed to the exclusion of all external stimuli. Zack is scheduled for an x-ray, blood test and possible surgical operation for a physical health problem.

---

1   **What is autism spectrum disorder (ASD)?**

A   Autism spectrum disorder is a severe, pervasive impairment in reciprocal socialization, qualitative impairment in communication and repetitive or unusual behaviour. The symptoms and severity of ASD vary greatly; two children with the same diagnosis may behave very differently and have strikingly different skills. In general, children with severe autism have significant impairments that include a marked inability to communicate with or interact with other people. Intelligence may or may not be impaired, so although most children with autism appear to gain new knowledge or skills slowly, and some affected children may show signs of intellectual disability, other children with autism have normal or above-average intelligence. The latter learn quickly, yet have difficulty communicating the information learnt to others verbally, applying what they know in everyday life and adjusting to social situations. A small number of children with autism are savants, meaning that they have exceptional skills in a specific area such as art, maths or music (Aylott 2000), but this is rare.

2 **What do you understand to be the cause of ASD?**

   (a) **Impaired genetic transmission.**
   (b) **Complications during pregnancy or birth.**
   (c) **Environmental factors.**
   (d) **Unknown or a combination of factors.**

A The answer is (d). There has been no specific cause identified for ASD and possible explanations implicate a combination of factors that might include all of the above. The incidence of ASD also appears to be higher in males.

3 **What is the prevalence of autism in the UK?**

A The prevalence in the UK is estimated at 1 in 100 (1 per cent), although this is not definitive as in some cases people on the autism spectrum may not be identified in childhood, particularly if the disorder is mild and there is little or no intellectual impairment. In such cases challenging behaviours are not displayed (Inglese and Elder 2009).

4 **What are the three impairments that are indicators of ASD?**

A Children with autism generally have problems in three crucial areas of development (Howlin and Asgharian 1999):

- social interaction
- social imagination
- flexible thinking.

The presentation of symptoms varies whereby some children show signs of autism in early infancy. Other children may develop normally for the first few months or years of life then either lose previously acquired language skills or suddenly become withdrawn or aggressive. These three areas may result in the following.

SOCIAL SKILLS

Children with autism will often make poor eye contact or avoid eye contact completely. They may not respond to voice and may appear not to hear at times. To their parents' dismay, they may be resistant to cuddling, holding or other physical contact, and they appear to be unaware of others' feelings. Children with autism can seem to prefer playing alone and may retreat into their own world. It is common that they will not ask for help or know how to take turns when playing with other children.

LANGUAGE

Speech development may be delayed or speech may be completely absent. Many children lose previously acquired ability to say words or sentences. When making requests the tone or rhythm of speech may be notably abnormal, and children may use a sing-song voice or robotic style of speech. Autism can cause children to be unable to start a conversation or maintain one started by someone else. They may repeat words or phrases verbatim, but with no understanding of their use or meaning. Indeed, they often do not appear to understand simple questions or directions.

BEHAVIOUR

A wide range of behaviours may be observed (Lecavalier 2006), including some of the following. Repetition is a common theme; for example, movements such as rocking, spinning or hand-flapping, Attempts to change specific behavioural routines or rituals are not well tolerated and may result in agitation at any disturbance or change of routine. Parents also report that their child moves around constantly. Many children with autism have specific or limited food preferences, eating only a small number of foods, or craving non-food items such as chalk or soil (a behaviour known as 'pica') (Ahearn et al. 2001). When having stories read to them, children on the autism spectrum are unlikely to point at pictures in the book and will notice even minor deviations from the story.

Children on the autism spectrum may also be fascinated by details, such as the spinning wheels of a toy car, but without demonstrating any understanding of the overall function of the wheels. A child with autism may be unusually sensitive to light, sound and touch, yet seem to be oblivious to pain. Young children with autism have difficulty sharing experiences with others and do not usually engage in imitative or make-believe play, which is crucial to later language and social development. Some will be overly compliant.

As they mature, some children with autism become more engaged with others and show fewer disturbances in behaviour. Children with the least severe problems may lead normal or near-normal lives. Others, however, continue to have difficulty with language or social skills, which has implications for developing friendships at school, and adolescence can exacerbate any existing behavioural problems.

Extra resource

Take some time to read the 'Ten things every child with autism wishes you knew' – a mother's perspective with practical advice (Notbohm 2012). There are key messages here for professionals and the public.

PRENATAL FACTORS THAT *MAY* CONTRIBUTE TO ASD

Antidepressant treatment during pregnancy, especially in the first 3 months, may be linked to ASD, as may nutritional deficiencies early in pregnancy, particularly insufficient folic acid intake. Older parents have a higher risk of having a baby with autism. Maternal infections or exposure to chemical pollutants such as metals and pesticides during pregnancy increase the risk, as do complications at or shortly after birth, including very low birth weight. However, the mechanism by which these factors might lead to autism is unclear (Gardener et al. 2009).

5 **Which professionals will be involved in establishing the diagnosis of ASD?**

A Presently, there is no medical test that can diagnose autism. Instead, specially trained mental health professionals and psychologists administer autism-specific behavioural evaluations. The sequence of events leading up to diagnosis is often precipitated by the parents who are often the first to notice that their child is showing unusual behaviour such as failing to make eye contact, not responding to his or her name or playing with toys in unusual, repetitive ways.

From birth to at least 3 years of age, every child should be screened for developmental milestones during routine health visitor and well-child clinic visits. When the health visitor or a parent raises concerns about a child's development, the doctor should refer the child to a specialist in child development and early intervention. A typical diagnostic evaluation involves a multidisciplinary team of professionals including paediatrician, psychiatrist, psychologist, speech and language therapist and child and adolescent mental health (CAMHS) services. Tests should include hearing, speech and language and an autism-specific screening tool such as the CHAT or M-CHAT (Child Autism Test or the Modified Child Autism Test). This type of comprehensive evaluation helps parents to understand as much as possible about their child's strengths and needs (Baron-Cohen et al. 2000).

Joanne finds it difficult to cope with Zack when she goes on shopping errands or in social situations as he becomes very difficult when anything new is introduced. The intensity of Zack's resistance to change appears to be increasing, and he has begun to demonstrate repetitive self-stimulatory behaviours such as rocking, spinning and flicking things on and off.

Most of his parents' anxiety is related to other people's reactions as Zack is perceived by strangers to be badly behaved and undisciplined.

Zack's health is generally good but he has been having repeated upper respiratory tract infections, ear infections, snoring and sleep problems. He has been referred to an ear, nose and throat specialist for assessment and possible surgical treatment for enlarged adenoids.

6   **What is the most significant challenge for Zack and his family when he has to attend appointments in primary, secondary and tertiary healthcare situations?**

(a) **Behaviour management and discipline.**
(b) **Zack's inability to cope with the concept of waiting his turn.**
(c) **Constant care and supervision.**
(d) **Zack's response to a new social situation and different sensory input.**
(e) **All of the above.**

A   The correct answer is (e). Zack's behaviour in response to any differences and changes in his usual routines will be stressors for his parents as well as for himself. Zack is likely to feel confusion and anxiety when he is faced with unfamiliar people, sights and sounds. Physical contact may also be difficult to tolerate, and, from his case history, he is overly sensitive to noise and reacts by covering is ears. He is unlikely to understand the concept of waiting and he may resort to self-stimulatory behaviours such as rocking or spinning.

Zack's parents may feel stress related to the acceptability of Zack's behaviour in the healthcare setting, particularly if he becomes hyperactive and difficult to control (Baker-Ericzen et al 2005; Hastings and Johnson 2001; Sanders and Morgan 1997). They may also experience anxiety, frustration and feelings of social isolation especially if they are not in touch with parents in similar circumstances (Boyd 2002; Hastings et al. 2005; Luther et al. 2005). It is imperative that Joanne and Paul are involved in Zack's management as they know the factors that increase his stress. Being consulted also increases their sense of control over events and conveys staff interest in their child's welfare. Contact with supportive family members and parents of other children with autism will help to decrease parental stress.

7   **How can Zack and his family be enabled to cope with his admission to hospital?**

(a) **Ascertain Zack's specific interests and needs before admission.**
(b) **Ascertain factors that help to reduce challenging behaviour situations.**
(c) **Prepare all staff in the department for Zack's arrival including such adjustments and modifications of the environment that can be made reasonably.**
(d) **Provide communication aids appropriate for Zack's specific individual needs.**
(e) **Ensure that his favourite toy or object is available to reduce his anxiety and behavioural distress.**
(f) **All of the above.**

A   The correct answer is (f), all of the above, of course. When a child with ASD needs to access the acute inpatient healthcare environment, modifications to the nursing plan of care are necessary. Some adjustments include working closely with his parents to understand better what strategies they need to employ to help Zack to deal with stressors. For example screening questions can be added to the initial nursing assessment that link parent strategies to identified challenges, recognizing how treatment interventions might be perceived differently by Zack and modifying the physical environment for safety.

Keys to success include understanding the core manifestations of Zack's impaired social interaction; problems with communication and repetitive and stereotypical patterns of behaviour and how the acute care environment will challenge those core symptoms. Children with ASD are more comfortable in familiar environments, and, therefore, preparation for tests and procedures ahead of time can greatly reduce Zack's anxiety. Although many children come to the inpatient ward as a result of an acute illness without time for a pre-admission visit, children with ASD who have scheduled pre-operative admissions could visit the inpatient unit as part of their pre-admission testing. Orientation to the outpatient and surgical units with nurses as well as play therapists could be included in this visit.

8   **How would you manage Zack's visit to the children's hospital for x-ray and venepuncture prior to inpatient treatment?**

A   You would conduct a pre-admission person-centred assessment with Zack's mother to ascertain the best way to approach him. Consider Zack's journey from arrival to discharge including giving consideration to the healthcare professionals who will be meeting Zack. Staff in the department should be made aware of his individual needs and the reasonable adjustments required for him, for example, appropriate language to use when speaking to Zack, his response to strangers including intolerance of proximity to others and direct physical contact.

If possible, a pre-admission visit to the hospital would help to ensure that disruption to his expected routine is minimized. In order to support Zack, his parents need preparatory information that they can read to him and show him pictures before his arrival in order to help him process the information prior to attending any healthcare setting. Photographs and symbols may also be useful as pictorial communication tools and social stories relating to the areas of the hospital that he will attend. A visual timetable of the blood test and x-ray procedures will help Zack and his family to understand the sequence of events. You would inform the radiography staff of his impending visit. A risk assessment should be conducted and equipment made available so that Zack can watch his Thomas the Tank Engine DVD to calm him down. Two nurses trained in therapeutic safe holding and autism should be present during the collection of blood samples.

9   **Which ONE of the following functions of play therapy would be most useful in helping a child on the autism spectrum?**

(a) **Stress relief.**
(b) **Modelling and rehearsing coping with unfamiliar events.**
(c) **Managing behavioural challenges arising from fear and anxiety.**
(d) **Psychological preparation for inpatient procedures.**

A   The correct answer is (c). Play is the ability to socialize, create and sustain interactive relationships with others in the world. It is the fundamental challenge that children on the autistic spectrum face and it is this relational deficit that results in so-called behavioural challenges. Research and policy guidelines have highlighted the importance of social development (National Institute for Health and Care Excellence (NICE) 2011; Vernon et al. 2012). It is upon this foundation that a child will more readily learn other desired skills such as self-help skills and cognitive skills.

Play is an excellent tool for helping children to move beyond the social barriers that accompany autism to shared interaction with other children and adults. Play therapy provides a dynamic approach to working with children that facilitates socialization and relationship-building. Play therapy with children on the autism spectrum still assumes a child-centred and child-led approach. The principles remain the same; the tools and techniques are simply adapted to meet the child's individuality and needs. Helping Zack to understand the meaning of some of his hospital experiences through toys, nurses and play specialists can help to reduce the stress that he experiences and to ensure a smoother transition in the case of future hospital visits.

10 **How can having a child with ASD affect families?**

A People are all different, and parents react individually to having a child with autism. Think for a while about how mothers, fathers, and siblings might respond; the stresses that they may feel; and the support that they may need. Much has been written about differing gender responses (Gray 2003; Hastings et al. 2001), about social isolation and support (Luther et al. 2005), coping styles (Hastings et al. 2005; Higgins et al. 2005; Mancil et al 2009) and the long-term impact on families (Gray 2002).

Activity

What do you think about the factors mentioned above and how these may affect families? Finish by looking at the guidance and information on two support sites: National Autistic Society UK (2015, http://www.autism.org.uk/living-with-autism/parents-relatives-and-carers.aspx) and Raising Children Network (Australia) (2015, http://raisingchildren.net.au/articles/autism_spectrum_disorder_family_stress.html).

Key points

- ASD is characterized by impairment in social interaction, social imagination and flexible thinking. It is manifested in lack of social skills, delayed and abnormal speech development, and a range of behaviours including repetition, rocking and limited and unusual food preferences.
- Behaviour management is a significant problem when a child with ASD needs to attend hospital for treatment. Thoughtful planning, collaboration with parents, and practical briefing of staff who will meet the child can reduce the child's stress, facilitate the completion of treatment, and set a positive precedent for future encounters.
- Play therapy has been shown to be an effective means of helping children with ASD to cope with hospital appointments and to communicate on their own terms with adults that they meet. An ASD pathway that includes play therapy is one way to routinize good practice in this area.

REFERENCES

Ahearn WH, Castine T, Nault K, Green G (2001) An assessment of food acceptance in children with autism or pervasive developmental disorder – not otherwise specified. *Journal of Autism and Developmental Disorders* 31: 505–511.

Aylott J (2000) Understanding children with autism: exploding the myths. *British Journal of Nursing* 9(12): 779–784.

Baker-Ericzen MJ, Brookman-Frazee L, Stahmer A (2005) Stress levels and adaptability in parents of toddlers with and without autism spectrum disorders. *Research and Practice for Persons with Severe Disabilities* 30: 194–204.

Baron-Cohen S, Wheelwright S, Cox A, Baird G, Charman T, Swettenham J, Doehring P (2000) Early identification of autism by Checklist for Autism in Toddlers (CHAT). *Journal of Royal Society of Medicine* 93(10): 521–525.

Boyd BA (2002) Examining the relationship between stress and lack of social support in mothers of children with autism. *Focus on Autism and Other Developmental Disabilities* 17: 208–215.

Gardener H, Spiegelman D, Buka SL (2009) Prenatal risk factors for autism: a comprehensive metaanalysis. *British Journal of Psychiatry* 195(1): 7–14 (DOI: 10.1192/bjp.bp.108.051672).

Gray DE (2002) Ten years on: A longitudinal study of families of children with autism. *Journal of Intellectual and Developmental Disability* 27: 215–222.

Gray DE (2003) Gender and coping: the parents of children with high functioning autism. *Social Science and Medicine* 56: 631–642.

Hastings RP, Johnson E (2001) Stress in UK families conducting intensive home-based behavioural intervention for their young child with autism. *Journal of Autism and Developmental Disorders* 31: 327–336.

Hastings RP, Kovshoff H, Brown T, Ward NJ, Espinosa FD, Remington B (2005). Coping strategies in mothers and fathers of preschool and school-aged children with autism. *Autism* 9: 377–391.

Higgins DJ, Bailey SR, Pearce JC (2005) Factors associated with functioning style and coping strategies of families with a child with an autism spectrum disorder. *Autism* 9: 125–137.

Howlin P, Asgharian A (1999) The diagnosis of autism and Asperger syndrome: findings from a survey of 770 families. *Developmental Medicine and Child Neurology* 41(12): 834–839.

Inglese MD, Elder JH (2009) Caring for children with autism spectrum disorder, part I: prevalence, etiology, and core features. *Journal of Pediatric Nursing* 24(1): 41–48.

Lecavalier L (2006) Behavioral and emotional problems in young people with pervasive developmental disorders: relative prevalence, effects of subject characteristics, and empirical classification. *Journal of Autism and Developmental Disorders* 36: 1101–1114.

Luther EH, Canham DL, Cureton VY (2005) Coping and social support for parents of children with autism. *The Journal of School Nursing* 21: 40–47.

Mancil GR, Boyd PA, Bedesem P (2009) Parental stress and autism: are there useful coping strategies? *Education and Training in Developmental Disabilities* 44(4): 523–537.

National Autistic Society (2015) *Parents, Relatives and Carers*. London: NAS. Available at: http://www.autism.org.uk/living-with-autism/parents-relatives-and-carers.aspx (accessed 25 January 2016).

National Institute for Health and Care Excellence (2011) *Autism Diagnosis in Children and Young People: Recognition, Referral and Diagnosis of Children and Young People on the Autism Spectrum*. Manchester: NICE.

Notbohm E (2012) *Ten Things Every Child with Autism Wishes you Knew (2nd edn)*. Reproduced by Autism Speaks. Available at: https://www.autismspeaks.org/sites/default/files/images/10_things.pdf (accessed 25 January 2016).

Raising Children Network (2015) *Autism Spectrum Disorder and Family Stress*. Victoria, Australia: RCN. Available at: http://raisingchildren.net.au/articles/autism_spectrum_disorder_family_stress.html (accessed 25 January 2016).

Sanders JL, Morgan SB (1997) Family stress and adjustment as perceived by parents of children with autism or Down syndrome: implications for intervention. *Child and Family Behavior Therapy* 19: 15–32.

Vernon TW, Koegel RL, Dauterman H, Stolen K (2012) An early social engagement intervention for young children with autism and their parents. *Journal of Autism and Developmental Disorders* 42(12): 2702–2717 (DOI:10.1007/s10803-012-1535-7).

A teenage girl with anorexia

Celeste Foster and Jane Benson

Case outline

Kim is a 13-year-old female who, until six months ago, could be described as a happy, academically bright young girl. Kim had commenced puberty and had begun menstruating, and had suffered with painful periods. As a result of this her mother took her to see her general practitioner (GP). The GP prescribed a preparation that could be bought over the counter, and advised Kim to eat healthily. Kim weighed 54 kg at this appointment.

Kim got straight on to the task of changing some of her eating habits. This included swapping treats such as chocolate and crisps for yoghurts and fruit. At the same time Kim joined a gymnastic club. She was especially successful at this. Her parents were proud of their daughter's achievements, and encouraged her new interest and mature approach. Her mother was the first of the parents to become concerned when she realized that her daughter was no longer menstruating. Her parents began noticing that she spent long periods in the bathroom, and that her friends were no longing calling at the house. They discussed this with Kim, who appeared dismissive, as if her parents were making 'a big deal out of nothing'.

A month later, the parents received a phone call from school asking them to meet the school nurse. The school nurse stated that Kim's grades were steadily deteriorating, also revealing that some of Kim's peers had reported that they had seen her throwing her lunch in the bin. The school nurse explained that she was worried about Kim's mood and that she was becoming a bit of a loner. It was suggested that the parents take Kim back to her GP for a check-up.

Her parents took Kim to the GP and were shocked by the information that the GP gave to them. In just a couple of months Kim had lost 9 kg: she now weighed 45 kg. Kim's physiological observations at this point were:

Blood pressure: 101/56
Pulse: 70
Temperature: 36°C, but she was wearing several layers of clothing.

The GP wanted to listen to Kim's chest. As Kim allowed the GP access for her stethoscope, the parents noticed Kim's protruding clavicle, and when allowing access to her back, the parents could see her protruding vertebrae. They were shocked and upset by this, but Kim did not seem to notice. The GP suggested that Kim should keep a food diary, took blood for tests and said that she would like to see her again in a week's time.

1   **What is a 'body mass index' and why is it more useful than just a weight?**

A   If we were told that a child's weight was 38 kg, it would not be possible to make an assessment of whether the child was under- or over-weight without access to other information such as their height, age and gender. Body mass index (BMI), which you came across in Case 1, is a measure of an individual's height to weight ratio, calculated using the specific formula below. It offers a clearer indicator of a child's relative weight. Body Mass Index is most useful when used in conjunction with a percentile growth chart (Royal College of Paediatrics and Child Health/Department of Health 2013). This plots the child's height and weight against the normal distribution within a national population of healthy children for a particular age and gender.

The threshold for diagnosis of anorexia nervosa is usually a BMI below 17.5 kg/m². However, in children it is also important to consider the interaction with the young person's expected development and the onset of puberty. Eating problems in children may show themselves as a failure to gain weight in expected growth periods, rather than weight loss. This can affect how quickly a parent or carer may notice their child's difficulties, as it is possible for children to become underweight for their height without weight loss (National Institute for health and Care Excellence [NICE] 2004).

Calculation exercise

The formula for calculating BMI is weight in kilograms/(height in metres)².

If Kim's height is 1.63 m, and weight is 45 kg, what is her BMI? A useful resource is the calculator at www.patient.co.uk/health/bmi-calculator.

The answer is given at the end of this case on p. 171.

2   **Kim is presenting with symptoms indicative of the early stages of development of an eating disorder. What are the characteristics of this condition?**

A   One or two of these characteristics may not signify the presence of disordered eating, but if a young person is presenting with a number of these signs it may indicate cause for concern.

- Weight loss, insufficient weight gain or growth relative to age.
- Intense fear of gaining weight.
- Changes to eating habits: avoidance of eating with others, secretive behaviour or obsessive relating to food.

- Mood swings, low or 'flat' mood.
- Dehydration, constipation, abdominal pains.
- Difficulty sleeping, fatigue, problems with concentration.
- Low blood pressure – feeling faint, dizziness.
- Downy hair on the body (can often see on nape of neck and arms) and loss of hair on the head.
- Feeling cold (due to poor blood circulation).
- Dry, rough skin.
- Loss of periods.
- Delayed puberty, or puberty halted once it has begun.
- Social withdrawal and isolation.
- Deterioration in school grades/performance.

(For further information refer to BEAT (2011) or visit www.b-eat.co.uk)

The term 'eating disorder' broadly refers to persistent changes in an individual's eating patterns that have a detrimental impact on their health and well-being. The two most common categories of eating disorders are bulimia nervosa and anorexia nervosa. Diagnosis of these conditions is made in accordance with the criteria defined in the 10th edition of the International Classification of Diseases (ICD 10, WHO 1992). In anorexia nervosa, the young person maintains a low weight through excessive control or restriction over their diet as a result of a preoccupation with body weight and shape. This is often expressed as a fear of fatness and weight gain or the pursuit of thinness. By contrast, bulimia nervosa describes a persistent pattern of binge eating and compensatory purging (vomiting or excessive laxative use), which is usually characterized by a feeling of loss of control. In both conditions, young people have a marked disturbance in their self-esteem and body image, and they can have underlying mood disorders such as depression (NICE 2004).

Kim's presentation fits with that of anorexia nervosa. This can affect men and women but is significantly more common in women, and the peak rate of onset is in the 13–19 age group. Some researchers have estimated that rates of anorexia nervosa in adolescence may be up to three times higher than in adulthood (Nicholls et al. 2011). It is estimated that between the peak ages of 15–19 years two girls in every thousand may be diagnosed with an eating disorder in the UK (Micali et al. 2013)

Anorexia nervosa is a complex condition, often lasting for many years. Long-term prognosis rates are variable, and in some cases can be very poor. The mortality rate in the population of people with an eating disorder is three times higher than for any other psychiatric disorder (NICE 2004). Early detection and treatment has an important part to play in influencing longer-term outcomes for individuals. Understanding the observable characteristic signs and symptoms of disordered eating in children and young people described above may help you to contribute to the nurse's role in early detection and intervention.

3 **What do you think are the contributing factors to the onset of anorexia nervosa in Kim's case? Think about the issues that concern most young people of her age and make a list of these. Think about how such ordinary concerns may have run out of control.**

A Many young people can experience what feels like a sudden change in body image with the onset of puberty. For girls this can be particularly around the hips, buttocks and abdomen. It is not unusual for young women to find that they are slightly above the expected height for weight ratio in the early stages of puberty. As in Kim's case the condition often starts with dieting behaviour that does not raise concern and that may actually bring reinforcing compliments from others (NICE 2004). It is part of a GP's role to promote a healthier lifestyle, including giving advice about changes to diet and exercise, and it is understandable that her parents inadvertently positively reinforced these messages, by praising the changes that Kim had made. Confusion over healthy eating advice has been identified as a specific contributing factor for eating disorders in young people (Treasure 2006). Once Kim had begun practising gymnastics she should have adapted her diet to match the calorie consumption of her training regime.

In the short term there may have been a perceived secondary gain for Kim, in that the weight loss would have caused her to stop menstruating, meaning no more painful and difficult to manage periods. Once there is significant weight loss, the effects of starvation have an impact upon a young person's ability to think clearly (Lask and Bryant-Waugh 2013). The perceived need to lose weight becomes paramount, with the individual unable to turn back without feeling like a failure or of losing control.

Other contributing factors that have been identified in the onset of an eating disorder include the experience of stressful or traumatic life events, societal and media pressures to be thin, a family history of eating problems and being temperamentally prone to perfectionism (Lask and Bryant-Waugh 2013).

Over the following week Kim loses a further kilogram. At this appointment the GP advises the family that she will refer Kim to the local CAMHS service. A plan is agreed with Kim and her parents. The GP continues to monitor Kim's weight and physical health on a weekly basis, the community CAMHS team sees Kim twice weekly, and Kim is no longer attending school.

---

4   **What does 'CAMHS' stand for?**

A   Child and Adolescent Mental Health Service; these services are organized along a pathway from primary care practitioners who a child would normally come across in everyday life, such as school nurses, through to specialist multidisciplinary community teams, and ultimately inpatient mental health services specifically for children and young people with severe and complex mental health problems. Individuals can move along this continuum according to where they are in their recovery. A specialist community CAMHS team is typically made up of child and adolescent psychiatrists, clinical child mental health nurses, clinical child psychologists and other psychological therapists, family therapists and social workers. These members of the team would all work collaboratively with the young person and their family to provide specialist assessment, diagnosis, formulation and implementation of psychological interventions, risk management and pharmacological treatment, as required. For more information about specialist CAMHS see NHS Choices (http://www.nhs.uk/pages/home.aspx) or My CAMHS choices (www.mycamhschoices.org).

Over the next month Kim loses more weight, and is referred to an inpatient CAMHS. When this service assesses Kim, her physical health is deteriorating. Her blood pressure is 80/50 and her temperature is 35.8°C. Kim has blue nail beds and dark circles around her eyes, which can be a clinical indicator of dehydration. Kim reports low mood and difficultly in concentrating. She is tearful throughout the assessment. Her weight is 36 kg and BMI is 13.7.

Kim is offered a place in the inpatient setting. Her parents accept the place, but Kim is reluctant, asserting that she could follow a plan of care at home and does not need to be admitted. As it is the first time that Kim has been admitted to a hospital and the first time that she has ever been away from her parents, she is distressed. The following day Kim takes fluids but will not eat anything.

5   **Outline the nursing care that Kim should receive in relation to the identified problems.**

A   In accordance with NICE (2004) clinical guidelines, nursing management of a young person with an eating disorder in an inpatient setting needs to have a focus on collaboration and engagement with the young person, and there should be a specific care plan. This should include the giving of appropriate information to the young person and their carers about the rationale for their care plan; risk assessment and management; appropriate support and supervision before, during and after mealtimes; and emotional and psychological support for the distress caused by re-feeding and separation from carers. For example, identifying enjoyable but low physical-impact distraction activities to undertake with the young person after meals can be an important and effective nursing intervention.

6   **This distraction activity is something that a student could undertake. Indeed, Kim might relate well to you. Think what you might do. What would be sufficiently enjoyable to distract Kim but not use up energy? Try to identify three possibilities.**

A   **IMPLEMENTING THE CARE PLAN**

Children experiencing symptoms of an eating disorder are usually highly anxious about any changes to their diet and routines, and they tend to demand a high level of attention to detail about all parts of their care plan as a means of trying to manage their fears. Because of this, they may seek to challenge or evade diet and treatment plans. The nursing team provides a vital role in maintaining boundaries, ensuring specific care plans are adhered to, and that all care is delivered with a high level of consistency. This way of working provides physical and emotional containment. It helps the young person to predict and engage with their treatment plan and can lessen distress and worries (Bakker et al. 2011).

Implementing the plan requires close liaison and partnership-working with the dietetic and medical team to ensure administration of a diet plan and prescribed medication to promote sustainable and safe weight gain. Without this, young people who have subjected themselves to excessive diet restriction or fasting are at high risk of developing a condition called re-feeding syndrome. This is characterized by electrolyte imbalance, cardiac arrhythmias, and, in worst cases, major organ dysfunction (Boateng et al. 2010).

Comprehensive assessment and close monitoring of physiological observations is required to manage the physical risks associated with:

- the complications of starvation
- physical complications of re-feeding or restoration of normal diet
- the complications of excessive exercise
- physical aspects of stunted or incomplete development
- physical complications of dietary imbalance such as a high fibre, low-fat diet.

Monitoring usually includes measuring weight, blood pressure and pulse, checking with regular blood tests, and making appropriate referrals for indicated investigations such as endocrinology and dual energy x-ray absorptiometry (DEXA) scans for early detection of irregularities in hormone levels and bone density.

The development of therapeutic relationships, including the identification of a key-worker or a core care team for both the young person and the family, is an essential contribution of nursing care to a young person's recovery (Lask and Bryant-Waugh 2013). Nurses monitor and support the young person and their family in relation to their identified mental health needs and risks. Nursing care is most effective when there is joint working between paediatric and mental health nurses.

Over the course of the next week Kim reduces her diet and fluid intake significantly, and repetitively states that if she could go home she would eat there, and get better. The team feels that Kim is getting worse, so a review meeting is called to discuss options. Kim's parents are clear that they do not wish to take her home. The decision is made that if Kim loses any more weight a nasogastric tube will need to be passed.

At this meeting, based on Kim's age and the severity of her condition, the decision is made in conjunction with her parents that if this procedure should become necessary the care team would be working in Kim's best interest, utilizing parental consent in accordance with the framework of The Children Act (1998, 2004) and national guidelines for seeking consent (Department of Health 2009).

With her parents present, Kim is made aware of all the issues that have been discussed in the meeting. She is informed about what will happen if she continues to lose weight. By the end of the week Kim has lost more weight, and the doctors again check with her parents that they still agree to a nasogastric tube being inserted. Once they confirm agreement, this is documented.

7 **Stop for a moment and reflect on the difficulty of working with Kim to improve her health, while also monitoring her for avoidance of the plan, and then treating her at her parents' consent against her own wishes.**

A Such complex situations are commonly faced by nurses, and it is vital to be clear on the rationale for decisions as well as the legal and ethical implications of actions. This requires striking a balance between acting in Kim's best interests and respecting her declared wishes. In this case the balance tips towards intervening against Kim's wishes, as to do nothing could lead to life-threatening deterioration. However, even in a situation as serious as this, the young person's preferences, choices and right to be involved in the decision-making process should still be promoted as much as possible. This requires skill in assessing whether or not Kim is able to make rational decisions about her treatment (competence), and in engagement and empowerment of Kim through formation of a therapeutic relationship.

The Best Interests Principle (General Medical Council 2007) provides practitioners with guidance when pondering the options that might be considered when making clinical decisions about a patient whose capacity to provide informed consent is diminished and who refuse to undergo a procedure. Those making the decision could consider the following aspects of the case.

- The treatment options that are clinically indicated in the particular case.
- The views of the child or young person, so far as they can express them, including any previously expressed preferences.
- The views of parents.
- The views of others close to the child or young person.
- The cultural, religious or other beliefs and values of the child or parents.
- The views of other healthcare professionals involved in providing care to the child or young person, and of any other professionals who have an interest in their welfare.
- Selecting the action that will least restrict the child or young person's future options.

8 **If you were the nurse passing the nasogastric tube, how would you prepare?**

A In any circumstance, the experience of having a nasogastric tube sited can be uncomfortable and can cause young people to feel anxious. However, for a young person with an eating disorder who fears above nearly all else losing control over what goes into their body, it can be an intensely distressing intervention and one to which they may be resistant. The requirement of the nurse in this situation is to maintain an empathic and compassionate position in terms of understanding and attending to the young person's concerns, while understanding that there is a duty of care to continue with and complete the procedure, despite their distress and sometimes vociferous protests. At the point at which a decision has been made that it is clinically indicated to undertake the procedure, it is also important for a young person to understand that negotiation regarding this is not an option available to them.

q   **Think this through. What will you need to do to reduce the physical unpleasantness and psychological distress as much as possible? Put yourself in Kim's place, but think also from the nurse's perspective.**

A   In addition to ensuring that you have appropriate training and supervision, and that you follow national and local clinical guidelines for the procedure, there are a number of other steps that can be helpful in these circumstances.

- Make sure that you have all the equipment prepared, in place and checked before you approach the young person to initiate the procedure. (Do a run through or a rehearsal of the procedure beforehand if needed, out of sight of the young person.)
- Talk the young person through the procedure, step by step, so that they know what to expect, demonstrating with the equipment.
- Be honest about the parts of the procedure that may feel a little uncomfortable, reassuring them that this is expected and that they are safe (for example: the eyes may water as the tube passes by the bridge of the nose; passing the tube down the back of the throat can activate the gag reflex).
- Encourage the young person to drink – directing them when to swallow in order to aid the passage of the tube.
- Once the procedure has been initiated it is important to proceed to completion (unless there are physical indicators that it is not safe to do so), even when the young person is protesting or upset. This can be difficult as a nurse, as it can feel as though it goes against caring principles. However, while stopping part way through a procedure may feel kinder in the moment, in the longer term it means only that the whole procedure will have to be repeated.

Caring for young people with eating disorders can exert a strong emotional impact upon nurses looking after the young people so there is a need to seek regular support and clinical supervision.

10   **Once Kim's urgent physical health needs have been addressed, and her weight has returned to within a safe range, what other evidence-based interventions might be helpful for Kim and her family?**

A   Treatment to support a young person's ongoing recovery continues long after discharge from inpatient care. The transition of care from the inpatient team to community services would usually occur through a multiprofessional discharge care planning meeting. Everyone involved in the case would be invited to that meeting, including the young person and their family. Identification of ongoing needs and decision-making about who is going to be responsible for specific components of the care plan are addressed at this meeting (Figure 19.1). The actions and agreements are minuted, often in the form of a care plan. An important part of the plan is the identification of a named person whose role is to coordinate multi-agency care and a regular review meeting. In the UK, a framework called the Care Programme Approach (CPA) is usually used for this (Department of Health 2008).

Evidence-based treatment and recovery plans for young people typically include ongoing support to adhere to the prescribed diet plan; psychoeducation; motivational enhancement; systemic family therapy; individual psychological therapy such as

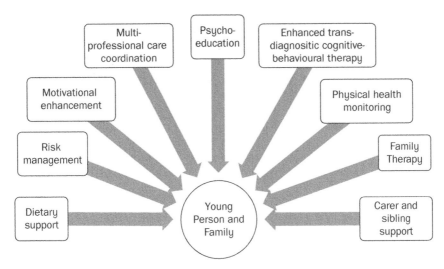

Figure 19.1 Multidisciplinary treatment plan

cognitive–behavioural therapy; support and educational work with carers; physical health monitoring and risk management (Dalle et al. 2013; Wolpert et al. 2006). The nature of the psychological therapies chosen will be influenced by patient preference, their motivation, the nature of associated psychological features of their condition, and their age or stage of development (NICE 2004).

Answer to calculation exercise

BMI = weight ÷ height^2 = 45 ÷ 1.63^2 = 45 ÷ 2.66 = 16.92 (Round up to BMI=17)

Key points

- Eating disorders are associated with particular developmental tasks in adolescence and difficulties achieving these, for instance separation and individuation, integrating physical changes of puberty into body image, identity development, peer and sexual relationship issues, and can be attempts at problem-solving in relation to these issues. Precipitating issues are often related to control, identity disturbance, coping with normal weight gain and fat re-distribution, and separation issues. Bullying, adverse life events and academic stress can also be potential triggers.
- Family/carer involvement in treatment is essential to recovery but must be balanced against the young person's emerging need for privacy and right to confidentiality. Carer strategies focus on empowering them to enforce boundaries confidently and to take control back from the eating disorder. Nurses should strive continuously to involve young people in their care even at times

when they have to take responsibility for safety and potentially having to intervene in ways with which the young person does not agree. There should be a focus on supportive, open-minded engagement.

- Skills in communication are essential for managing confidentiality; challenging stigma; supporting siblings so that they do not feel marginalized; giving information to carers; and addressing safeguarding issues. It is essential that the multidisciplinary team works alongside the young person to fight the eating disorder through consistent and predictable care (Golan 2013). Multiprofessional care coordination and preparing and supporting the family to maintain progress at home are vital factors for success.

REFERENCES

Bakker R, van Meijel B, Beukers L, van Ommen J, Meerwijk E, van Elburg A (2011) Recovery of normal body weight in adolescents with anorexia nervosa: the nurses' perspective on effective interventions. *Journal of Child and Adolescent Psychiatric Nursing* 24(1):16–22.

BEAT (2011) *Caring for a Child or Adolescent with an Eating Disorder*. Norwich: BEAT/The Rank Foundation. Available at: www.b-eat.co.uk (accessed 25 January 2016).

Boateng A, Sriram K, Meguid M, Crook M (2010) Re-feeding syndrome: treatment considerations based on collective analysis of literature case reports. *Nutrition* 26(2): 156–167.

Dalle Grave R, Calugi S, Doll HA, Fairburn CG (2013) Enhanced cognitive behaviour therapy for adolescents with anorexia nervosa: an alternative to family therapy? *Behaviour Research and Therapy* 51(1): R9–R12.

Department of Health (2008) *Refocusing the Care Programme Approach: Policy and Positive Practice Guidance*. London: Published by COI for The Department of Health. Available at: http://webarchive.nationalarchives.gov.uk/20130107105354/http://www.dh.gov.uk/prod_consum_dh/groups/dh_digitalassets/@dh/@en/documents/digitalasset/dh_083649.pdf (accessed 25 January 2016).

Department Health (2009) *Reference Guide to Consent for Examination or Treatment (2nd edn)*. London: Department of Health. Available at: https://www.gov.uk/government/publications/reference-guide-to-consent-for-examination-or-treatment-second-edition (accessed 25 January 2016).

General Medical Council (2007) *0-18yrs Guidance for All Doctors*. Manchester: General Medical Council.

Golan M (2013) The journey from opposition to recovery from eating disorders: multidisciplinary model integrating narrative counseling and motivational interviewing in traditional approaches. *Journal of Eating Disorders* 1(1): 19.

Lask B, Bryant-Waugh R (eds) (2013) *Eating Disorders in Childhood and Adolescence*. Hove: Routledge.

Micali N, Hagberg KW, Petersen I, Treasure JL (2013) The incidence of eating disorders in the UK in 2000–2009: findings from the General Practice Research Database. *BMJ Open* 3(5): e002646 (DOI:10.1136/bmjopen-2013-002646).

National Institute for Health and Care Excellence (2004) *Eating Disorders. Core Interventions in the Treatment and Management of Anorexia Nervosa, Bulimia Nervosa and related Eating Disorders (NICE Clinical Guideline 9)*. London: NICE www.nice.org.uk/cg9 (accessed 25 January 2016).

Nicholls D, Lynn R, Viner RM (2011) Childhood eating disorders: British National Surveillance Study. *British Journal of Psychiatry* 198: 295–301.

Royal College of Paediatrics and Child Health/Department of Health (2013) *UK Growth Charts (2nd edn)*. London: RCPCH.

Treasure J (2006) *Anorexia Nervosa: A Survival Guide for Families, Friends and Sufferers*. Hove: Routledge.

Wolpert M, Fuggle P, Cottrell D, et al. (2006) *Drawing on the Evidence: Advice for Mental Health Professionals Working with Children and Adolescents (2nd edn)*. London: CAMHS Publications.

World Health Organization (1992) *International Classification of Diseases*. Geneva: WHO. Available at: http://www.who.int/classifications/icd/en/ (accessed 25 January 2016).

Sickle cell disease

Janice Grant and Tracey Bloodworth

Case outline

Shola is a 7-year-old girl of Nigerian parentage who has sickle cell disease and has been admitted to a children's hospital with a chest infection. She is feverish with a temperature of 38.5°C, rapid respirations, difficulty breathing and chest pain associated with prolonged coughing. She is accompanied by her mother Lakesia.

Shola's sickle cell disease was diagnosed when she was 6 years old soon after she arrived in the UK with her 25-year-old mother. Her mother is a single parent and the whereabouts of her father is unknown after he left the family six months ago. The family is in temporary accommodation with no social support, and Lakesia has two other children aged 5 and 2 years. Both of Shola's younger siblings have been tested and are carriers of the sickle cell disease trait (HbAS).

Lakesia's English is limited but she tells the admitting nurse that Shola has not had her prescribed prophylactic antibiotics regularly as she sometimes forgets to request the repeat prescription or is unable to collect it as she has no childcare. The nurse caring for Shola notices that her conjunctiva are yellow, she is very lethargic and appears to be small for her age. Shola is complaining of pain in her knees, and her mother states that she still wets the bed, which Shola finds particularly embarrassing.

Shola has had several previous admissions for sickle cell crises, and her ongoing care and management are usually managed by the staff in the children's haematology centre.

Baseline observations on admission

Temperature: 38.5°C
Pulse: 120 bpm
Blood pressure: 110/60
SpO_2: 94%
Weight: 12 kg

1 **What is sickle cell disease?**

(a) **A type of blood cancer.**
(b) **An autosomal recessive genetic disorder of the red blood cells.**
(c) **A disease of the joints.**
(d) **A fatal disease that cannot be treated.**

A The correct answer is (b). Sickle cell disease is the result of a recessively inherited genetic condition caused by a mutation of the ß haemoglobin gene leading to the formation of abnormal haemoglobin. Sickle haemoglobin (HbS) is insoluble when deprived of oxygen, resulting in the formation of long polymers. These polymers damage the red blood cell membranes causing them to distort into rigid sickle or crescent shapes. The sickle-shaped cells are less robust and have reduced oxygen-carrying capacity, which in turn leads to red blood cell breakdown (haemolysis), oxygen deprivation, anaemia, vaso-occlusion, pain, risk of serious infections and damage to vital organs. Sickle cell disease occurs when the child has the homozygous condition (HbSS) where genes are inherited from both parents, while the heterozygous state (HbAS) is defined as sickle cell trait. Sickle cell disease is common in Africa, India and Arabia, whereas the trait is common around the Mediterranean and in North Americans of mixed heritage. Males and females are affected with equal frequency.

INHERITING THE DISEASE

As shown in Table 20.1, if both parents carry the trait each pregnancy carries a 25 per cent chance that the child will have normal haemoglobin (HbAA), a 50 per cent chance that they will have the heterozygous sickle cell trait (HbAS) and 25 per cent chance that the child will have sickle cell disease (HbSS). Sickle cell disease (HbSS genotype) occurs if HbS is transmitted from each parent.

Table 20.2 shows that if one parent is HbSS and the other is HbAS then each pregnancy has a 50 per cent chance of having a child with sickle cell disease and a 50 per cent chance of having a child with the heterozygous sickle cell trait.

The final possibility is that one parent is HbAA (normal) and the other is HbSS. In this case, all of the children will have the sickle cell trait, none will have completely normal haemoglobin, and none will have sickle cell disease (Table 20.3).

Table 20.1 Mode of inheritance if both parents have the heterozygous gene for sickle cell disease

Father with sickle cell trait HbAS		*Mother with sickle cell trait HbAS*	
AA child unaffected	**SA** child with the sickle cell trait	**SA** child with the sickle cell trait	**SS** child with sickle cell disease

A, normal gene; **S**, sickle cell gene.

Table 20.2 Mode of inheritance if one parent is heterozygous and the other homozygous for sickle cell disease

Father with sickle cell trait Hb**AS**		Mother with sickle cell disease Hb**SS**	
AS child with the sickle cell trait	**SS** child with sickle cell disease	**AS** child with the sickle cell trait	**SS** child with sickle cell disease

A, normal gene; **S**, sickle cell gene.

Table 20.3 Mode of inheritance if one parent has normal haemoglobin and the other has the homozygous gene for sickle cell disease

Unaffected father Hb**AA**		Mother with sickle cell trait Hb**SS**	
AS child with the sickle cell trait	**AS** child with the sickle cell trait	**AS** child with the sickle cell trait	**AS** child with the sickle cell trait

A, normal gene; **S**, sickle cell gene.

2 **Sickle cell disease is a hereditary long-term disorder. What is the *most* usual cause of serious illness and sometimes death?**

(a) **Acute chest syndrome.**
(b) **Enlarged spleen.**
(c) **Hypokalaemia.**
(d) **Sickling crisis.**

A The correct answer is (a). Acute chest syndrome is a serious complication of sickle cell disease, the exact cause of which is unknown, but it is thought that since the lungs are already damaged by the underlying disease an infection in the lungs further impairs gaseous exchange resulting in a life-threatening lung condition. Children with acute chest syndrome usually present with upper respiratory tract infections, chest pain, cough, dyspnoea and tachypnoea. They are referred to hospital as a medical emergency if they have a fever, respiratory distress or increasing hypoxia as assessed by SpO$_2$ readings. The increasing hypoxia results in a vicious cycle of worsening hypoxia and vaso-occlusion that requires immediate treatment with antibiotics, analgesics, blood transfusion, humidified oxygen and rehydration with intravenous fluids. Lifelong prophylactic antibiotics are prescribed for children with this disorder in an effort to prevent chest infections occurring, but may become ineffective if the medication is not taken as prescribed. Rees et al. (2010) warn of the need for more research in the field of long-term health complications for those with sickle cell disease. The situation is complex and often unpredictable.

3 **In order to stabilize Shola's acute chest syndrome and prevent it becoming more critical, which of the following is the *most* important intervention?**

(a) **Intravenous fluid infusion.**
(b) **Bed rest.**

(c) **Chest physiotherapy.**
(d) **Blood transfusion and oxygen therapy.**

A   The correct answer is (d). A blood transfusion is given to reduce the percentage of sickled red blood cells in circulation and to increase the number of red blood cells that are available to carry a normal complement of oxygen. Oxygenation of all tissues (including the lungs themselves) will be further improved by the administration of oxygen therapy.

4   **What are the most serious indicators that a child with sickle cell disease requires urgent nursing and medical interventions?**

(a) **Joint pain, no fever or lethargy.**
(b) **Joint pain with high fever.**
(c) **Cough, breathlessness and fever.**
(d) **Abdominal pain and jaundice.**

A   The correct answer is (c). Although all the above are indicators of illness in a child with sickle cell disease, respiratory infection is the commonest cause of death in children with sickle cell disease, and acute chest syndrome or crisis is a life-threatening condition.

Clinically, children with sickle cell disease present with a haemolytic type of anaemia and are affected by sickle cell crises occurring at varying frequency. Crises are caused by acute sickling of the cells resulting in bleeding, pooling of blood in the spleen, and occlusion of arteries. The pain associated with crises requires effective intervention (Maxwell et al. 1999). Crises are characterized as one of the following.

- *Haemolytic anaemic crisis*: acute sickling causing anaemia that is usually accompanied by painful crises.
- *Painful vascular occlusive crisis*: this is caused by occlusions within the arteries supplying bones (hips, shoulders and vertebrae), the lungs and the spleen. The most serious crises can occur in the central nervous system and the spinal cord. They are precipitated by infection, dehydration, cold, de-oxygenation, and vigorous exercise.
- *Aplastic crisis*: this is usually caused by infection with parvovirus (slapped cheek syndrome) and presents as a particularly severe anaemia.
- *Visceral sequestration crisis*: this type of crisis is caused by sickling within organs resulting in pooling of blood in the affected organ with serious anaemia. A severe chest infection can be a common and fatal cause of visceral sequestration crisis.
- *Hand-foot syndrome*: sickling of the red blood cells can cause painful swelling of the hands and feet (dactylitis) as blood vessels become blocked. Although painful, no damage is caused, and the condition often resolves in one to four weeks with treatment.

Complications of sickle cell disease include stroke, transient ischaemic attacks, splenic sequestration crisis (usually seen in children aged between 6 months and 3 years), renal hypertension (De Gracia-Nieto et al. 2011), pulmonary hypertension, bone necrosis, osteomyelitis, enlarged spleen (splenomegaly) and chronic liver disease.

5   **What would be the most important observations that the nurse assigned to Shola should monitor?**

  (a) **Pain scores.**
  (b) **Heart rate and blood pressure.**
  (c) **Oxygen saturation.**
  (d) **State of hydration and fluid balance chart.**

A   The correct answer is (c). All the above measurements are important and would be taken at frequent intervals as they provide information on Shola's condition on an ongoing basis. Parameters from physiological observations are part of many early warning scoring systems. However, it is especially important to monitor oxygen saturation via pulse oximetry as low oxygen saturation can precipitate a sickling crisis, and Shola is already compromised by her chest infection and acute chest syndrome crisis. Pain scores and administration of prescribed analgesia are also an important part of Shola's care and management.

6   **Which of the following professionals will be involved with Shola's ongoing health, psychological and social care in the community?**

  (a) **Social worker and general practitioner (GP).**
  (b) **School health advisor and health visitor.**
  (c) **School teacher and classroom assistant.**
  (d) **Occupational therapist.**

A   The correct answer is (a). It is essential that Shola takes her prescribed penicillin to prevent pneumococcal infections, and the social worker will work with Lakesia to ensure that she collects the medications prescribed by the GP on a regular basis. The social worker will also be involved in liaison with the local authority in providing help and assistance with housing and information on social provision. Support for families comes from many sources such as the specialist members of clinical staff from the haemophilia hospital team, community team, counsellors, health visitor, teachers, family, GP and church groups. It is important for the family to gain trust in support networks and to feel able to discuss any concerns that may arise. Community medical support for children with sickle cell disease is crucial (Brousse et al. 2014).

7   **Why might bedwetting be a problem, and which professionals will help with its management?**

A   Shola has reported episodes of bedwetting (nocturnal enuresis) which is a common occurrence in children with sickle cell disease as a result of glomerular hyper-filtration, damage to the kidneys by the 'stickiness' of the blood, and the need to drink large quantities of fluid to prevent dehydration. Most children affected by this problem experience only nocturnal enuresis, but daytime 'accidents' can also occur. Enuresis may have a potentially negative impact on Shona, particularly if she has an episode during the day at school. The health visitor will be involved in providing an enuresis alarm and explaining how this can be part of the management plan.

  Bedwetting and daytime enuresis may have a psychological impact on Shola. For example, she may be embarrassed because she either smells of urine or is worried about incidents at school. She will be unable to engage in sleepovers with school friends or to participate in school trips, although this can be overcome in the short term by the administration of the synthetic version of the anti-diuretic hormone called desmopressin. School friends or teachers may notice the smell of urine, and if Lakesia cannot afford to heat water for Shola to bathe every morning, Shola may become self-conscious about her personal hygiene.

In relation to management of Shola's enuresis at home, Lakesia would be advised to limit fluid intake after 7 pm (as long as Shola has had good intake during the day). Lakesia would be advised to ensure that the process of 'double micturition' (use of the toilet once and then again five minutes later) is used prior to Shola going to bed. The mother may also find it helpful to take Shola to use the toilet at bedtime and a few hours later. Alarms do not always work for this client group, but community enuresis clinics can be helpful with support and advice. Provision for children with sickle cell disease includes a dedicated clinical psychologist who can work with families on a range of issues such as pain control, distraction techniques, needle phobia, compliance issues and cognitive testing.

The hospital social worker is an excellent resource for families with a long-term condition to assist them with financial, immigration and housing issues. The community social worker may be able to help Lakesia to identify sources of extra finance for help with washing Shola's bedding every day as she may not have a washing machine at home. There may also be perceived social stigma attached to awareness of the problem if neighbours see bed sheets drying on a washing line all the time.

The health visitor is also pivotal in helping Lakesia to access childcare support (for example, a Sure Start centre) for help with parenting and social contact. Free nursery provision for at least some time would be helpful to give Lakesia some help with the younger children and to improve her ability to cope with her child with a long-term condition.

8 **What can be done to promote a positive school experience for Shola?**

A Before starting any formal education and during her school years, Shola's mother has a responsibility to inform the nursery and school that Shola has this disorder and is unable to participate in vigorous activities, and also that she may be tired and lethargic because of chronic low haemoglobin. Furthermore, the school health advisor is able to advise teachers and classroom assistants on the specific requirements such as the need for Shola to drink frequently to avoid dehydration, to participate in physical activities, have rest periods, and be able to meet the necessity for frequent visits to the toilet.

Although sickle cell disease has no effect on intelligence, Shola may find it difficult to concentrate when she is in pain, or she may become tired and lethargic if her chronic anaemia is severe. Shola may have to miss lessons or take days off school for clinic attendance during and after a crisis. Frequent or prolonged interruptions from school may cause Shola to fall behind with her school work. If this is the case, Lakesia can help by ensuring that the teachers understand Shola's medical condition thus helping her to keep up with lessons. This may require that Shola always has some work that can be done at home if she is away from school for extended periods. The teacher will need a letter of permission from Lakesia so that she will be contacted at the first indication of even mild sickle cell pain and that Shona is excused from strenuous exercise. This information has to be reiterated every time Shola moves to a different class.

9 **How are physical and psychological health promotion addressed?**

A The health visitor and the outpatient haematology clinic staff will ensure that Shona receives all her immunizations according to the schedule (Public Health England 2015), and at the age of 7 she should be up to date with routine vaccinations. In addition, the following vaccines should be given to prevent avoidable infections (NICE 2010):

- pneumococcus vaccine, with regular boosters at least every five years
- influenza vaccine every autumn
- haemophilus influenzae type b (Hib)
- meningitis C (Men C).

Dietary supplements such as folic acid once per day are recommended to help in the manufacture of red blood cells. Shola's home environment should be warm, clean, free from draughts, damp and mould in order to reduce the risk of infection and avoid stressors that may contribute to physical and psychological ill health. This may not be easy for Lakesia as a single mother in her current social situation, and a social worker may be able to provide support with ensuring that any social support needed to achieve this is secured. The health visitor will also intervene to support the case for additional heating or better housing.

10 **How might compliance change as Shola moves through childhood?**

A Some younger children refuse their medication as a means of assuming personal control and autonomy. Reward charts and stickers, talking about the disease, and gaining the trust of the child can help with compliance. As children with sickle cell disease get older, attending clinics, conferences and special patient group days will help them to realize that they are not alone and can lead a near-normal lifestyle if they look after themselves.

Problems with compliance usually affect older children with sickle cell disease, which is often manifested by denial of their condition. As part of their normal development adolescents often think they are invincible, refuse medication and feel they can drink alcohol and smoke regardless of their physical limitations in order to maintain peer group relationship. School refusal is not common, but adolescents may complain of tiredness and difficulty getting up in the morning, feeling victimized when they are unable to perform well in physical education lessons, and lack of understanding from peers and teachers can cause upset. The role of effective communication and support including from other sickle cell disease sufferers must not be underestimated.

The unpredictability of the disease process often causes the most disruption, distress and upset to the families as it is difficult for them to plan ahead and events such as holidays or engaging with peers in normal childish pursuits become a major challenge. However, there remains hope for effective interventions for sickle cell disease, with potential for new treatments always arising (Stuart and Nagel 2004).

Extra resource

Read about new treatments that are emerging by going to the Sickle Cell Society web pages on research (http://sicklecellsociety.org/resource-type/research-report/).

Key points

- Sickle cell disease is a recessively inherited genetic condition characterized by mis-shaped red blood cells carrying abnormal haemoglobin and limited oxygen-carrying capacity.
- Respiratory infection and acute chest syndrome are the most dangerous facets of life with sickle cell disease, although crises caused by sickling of the cells can be painful, debilitating and dangerous.
- Normal health promotion interventions are vital to preventing additional problems, together with immunizations (particularly against respiratory infection). Families often require the support of schools, GP, social worker and other services to deal with the many problems that can develop.

REFERENCES

Brousse V, Makani J, Rees DC (2014) Management of sickle cell disease in the community. *British Medical Journal* 348: 1–9.

De Gracia-Nieto AE, Samper AO, Rojas-Cruz C, Gascon LG, Sanjuan JB, Mavrich HV (2011) Genitourinary manifestations of sickle cell disease. *Archivos Españoles de Urología* 64(7): 597–604.

Maxwell K, Streetly A, Bevan D (1999) Experiences of hospital care and treatment seeking for pain from sickle cell disease: qualitative study. *BMJ* 318(7196): 1585–1590. Available at: http://www.ncbi.nlm.nih.gov/pmc/articles/PMC28137/ (accessed 26 January 2016).

National Institute for Health and Care Excellence (2010) *Sickle Cell Disease: Prevention of Complications of Sickle Cell Disease (Clinical knowledge Summaries)*. London: NICE. Available at: http://cks.nice.org.uk/sickle-cell-disease#!scenario:3 (accessed 26 January 2016).

Public Health England (2015) *Complete Immunisation Schedule*. London: PHE. Available at: https://www.gov.uk/government/uploads/system/uploads/attachment_data/file/473570/9406_PHE_2015_Complete_Immunisation_Schedule_A4_21.pdf (accessed 26 January 2016).

Rees DC, Williams TN, Gladwin MT (2010) Sickle-cell disease. *Lancet* 376(9757): 2018–2031.

Sickle Cell Society (2014) *Research Reports*. Available at: http://sicklecellsociety.org/resource-type/research-report/ (accessed 26 January 2016).

Stuart MJ, Nagel R L (2004) Sickle cell disease. *Lancet* 364: 1343–60.

PART 7
Life-Limiting Conditions and Palliative Care

Deterioration of mobility in a boy with Duchenne muscular dystrophy

Tony Long and Fran Binici

Case outline

John is a 10-year-old boy who has Duchenne muscular dystrophy. At his clinic appointment it has become clear to the health team that his mobility has started to decline and additional problems are emerging. The report from the cardiologist indicates a degree of impending heart failure, while x-ray assessment suggests the possibility of a vertebral fracture. The physiotherapy assessment shows steady reduction in ambulatory ability, although this is not confirmed by John's parents. John readily admits that he refuses to wear ankle splints as often as he should. The parents have reported, however, that John's behaviour has become challenging sometimes and that he seems to have mood swings occasionally.

---

1 **What is Duchenne muscular dystrophy?**

A Duchenne muscular dystrophy, usually abbreviated to DMD, is a neuromuscular condition caused by lack of the protein dystrophin. There are many more forms of muscular dystrophy, but DMD is by far the most common. It is characterized by progressive muscle weakness in the proximal muscles (not so much those involved in fine movement of the hands and fingers until much later in the condition). It occurs almost always in boys: about 1 in 3,500. You read about Mendelian inheritance in Case 20 (on sickle cell disease). In this case, the inheritance is X-linked (the DMD gene residing on the X chromosome). Boys have one X and one Y chromosome, so if the faulty X chromosome is inherited from a carrier mother, they will have the disease. (See Figure 21.1) Since girls have two X chromosomes they are usually spared although they may be a carrier. The normal gene on the other X chromosome compensates for the faulty one. However, in perhaps half of cases of DMD there is not an inherited fault in the parent. There is a spontaneous mutation in the DNA of the egg from which the pregnancy resulted, leading to the boy having DMD. However, the risk of having further boys affected by the condition is reduced.

The mechanism of the disease is that the DMD gene for making dystrophin is faulty. Dystrophin is a protein located mostly in the skeletal muscles (used for movement) and in cardiac muscle. It is part of a protein complex (a group of interacting proteins) that help to bind muscle cells together and to strengthen muscle fibres. It also protects

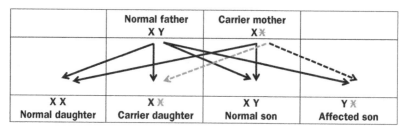

Figure 21.1 Duchenne muscular dystrophy genetic inheritance

muscles from injury. Lack of dystrophin, then, leads to damage of the muscle fibres and consequent weakening of the muscle. There is no cure for DMD. It is important to note that the dystrophin protein is also found within the brain. A significant proportion of boys with DMD will also have a degree of learning and behavioural difficulties that do not grow worse over time but need to be recognized to ensure appropriate management.

2   **What problems are caused by DMD?**

A   Since any muscle tissue can be affected, the effects are widespread through the body, and the side effects of treatment can impose additional problems. Steroids are used to treat DMD as they have been found to be beneficial in slowing down the disease process for approximately two years. The steroids used are either prednisolone or deflazacort given either daily or on a ten days on, ten days off regime. Regardless, the cost is significant side effects. Currently, a research trial called FOR DMD is being conducted to compare these medicines and regimes

THE MUSCLES INVOLVED IN MOVEMENT

Activity

Watch the Duchenne Foundation Australia You Tube video (2014, https://www.youtube.com/watch?v=AF4D4TyE9NM) demonstrating Gower's sign, a compensatory technique adopted by affected children to move from lying to standing.

Perhaps the most obvious site of muscular degeneration is in the muscles of the legs, hips and shoulders. This is demonstrated clearly in the classic manifestation of Gower's sign as the child adopts the technique of climbing up his own legs.

THE MUSCLES INVOLVED IN POSTURE

Posture is maintained partly by the spinal muscles and by the muscles of the shoulder girdle, the pelvis and the neck. Contracture of muscles, and sometimes unbalanced forces as one muscle become weaker than another in one of these groups, causes stiffness and reduction in the range of movement. A common problem in DMD is contracture at the ankle joint and tightening of the Achilles tendon, leading to a toe-down foot position that seriously limits the ability to stand and walk. Scoliosis of the spine is common, especially if steroid treatment is not instigated, due to asymmetrical contractures and persistently poor posture.

In John's case, physiotherapy assessment has identified gradual decline in function. That the family does not hold the same perspective may be partially because of the insidious nature of the decline and partly as a result of reluctance to accept such a terrible truth. John has been encouraged to wear night splints to help to promote better foot posture to maintain a stable base for walking. John admits that he is not using the splints, and his parents feel unable to enforce the use of them as he 'just takes them off'. The benefits and consequences of using or not using splints is discussed, and then it is for John and his parents to decide.

HEART MUSCLE

The heart itself is made up mostly of muscle, and this, too, is affected by DMD, eventually leading to cardiomyopathy (weakening of the heart muscle with consequent deterioration in function). The spaces in the heart grow larger, while the muscle wall of the ventricles can become thinner. In DMD the heart is monitored every two years up to the age of 10 and then yearly thereafter. In ultrasound, fraction shortening values relate to the change in left ventricular diameter between the relaxed and contracted states – a measure of cardiac function. When the measurements begin to reduce then cardiac medication is instigated to help to improve or maintain heart function. Cardiac assessment is then undertaken more frequently. John has had a recent assessment with the cardiologist that indicated that his cardiac function is impaired and there is a need for further assessment with a view to starting medication.

RESPIRATORY MUSCLES

Respiration relies upon the diaphragm and intercostal muscles (aided by ancillary muscles in the shoulders when struggling for breath). As these muscles are affected by DMD, although usually only once the ability to walk is lost, breathing and coughing become less effective, introducing greater risk of infection. So far, John is not troubled by respiratory problems, but this, too, needs to be monitored and managed. At each clinic appointment John's respiratory effort is assessed through spirometry. Polysomnography records oxygen saturation, heart and respiratory rate, eye movement, body position, muscle electrical activity and electroencephalogram (EEG) during sleep. Polysomnography studies will be carried out when clinical assessment of John's respiratory ability indicates the need so that appropriate intervention can be instigated.

SIDE EFFECTS OF STEROID THERAPY

Height tends to be stunted with steroid therapy, while increase in weight is stimulated (steroids increase appetite). A further issue with development is that puberty is usually delayed, and this may be upsetting for the boy. Diabetes may ensue since food metabolism is affected, with fewer calories required (despite the increased appetite) and insulin resistance is encountered. Cataracts may develop. Bone demineralization is a common side effect of steroid therapy, and, when combined with poor posture from atrophy of the spinal muscles, this can lead to fractures of the vertebrae. John has been on steroids for five years and is seen in the clinic on a six-monthly basis to monitor the benefits and risks of taking this medication. He is also known in other specialist departments in the hospital that assess and manage complications associated with his condition and steroid use.

3   **How is DMD diagnosed?**

A   Although the problem is present from birth, symptoms may not become noticeable until the second or third year or even later. Often, parents will be concerned about the child's gait, describing a waddling style of walking, and will report unexpected difficulty in climbing stairs or in running and jumping. They may appear to be clumsy, often falling. This is sometimes in conjunction with a delay in cognitive ability.

Three tests are used to explore the diagnosis. A blood test for creatine kinase (an enzyme produced by the breakdown of muscle tissue) will show from 10 to 100 times the normal value, which is indicative of muscle damage. If this is elevated and DMD is suspected because of the history taken and clinical examination, then DNA testing for DMD is performed looking for a deletion or duplication in the gene sequencing. If a definitive diagnosis cannot be made from DNA testing then a muscle biopsy will be considered. A muscle biopsy is usually taken from the thigh – one of the muscles particularly affected by DMD. This is examined through a number of techniques to discover the abnormal muscle structure due to the missing dystrophin. You can read more about this in a publication from the Muscular Dystrophy Campaign (2008). If the expected abnormality is found, a further blood test may be performed to identify the faulty DMD gene.

The North Star Ambulatory Assessment (North Star Clinical Network 2014) was developed by a network of senior specialist clinicians from DMD treatment centres across the UK. The assessment grades activity according to the degree of independence and modification made to normal technique to achieve the activity or task. Adaptations to activity are necessary because of the underlying progressive muscular weakness.

2 = No obvious modification of the activity.
1 = Activity achieved through modification but independent of others' physical assistance.
0 = Unable to complete the activity independently.

Each time John attends the DMD/steroid clinic he undertakes the North Star Assessment and this helps the clinicians and therapist to assess his ability to carry out the specific tasks. This assessment, in conjunction with what is reported by the child and parents, is used to determine the impact of DMD at each visit and to plan for any interventions that are required.

PROBLEMS AND INTERVENTIONS IN DIFFERENT AGE GROUPS

Although the precise ages differ for the occurrence of these changes, there are stages that differ in terms of the nature of problems presenting and the treatment provided. An internationally agreed guide for parents suggests the following stages (Bushby et al. 2010a,2010b; Treat-NMD 2011).

Pre-symptomatic stage

Unless there is a family history of DMD, boys are not usually diagnosed at this stage. Parents may recognize subtle signs retrospectively.

Early ambulatory stage

Diagnosis is most likely to be made at this stage. Classic signs of DMD arise, including Gower's sign and waddling gait. A physiotherapy exercise regime may be introduced to prevent joint stiffness. Since motor skills are still developing, steroid therapy will be discussed and may be commenced once motor ability appears to level off: usually between the ages of 4 and 6 years. Heart and breathing problems would not be expected at this stage. However, surveillance of cardiac and respiratory function is maintained routinely. Cardiac assessment is undertaken every two years until the age of 10, or more frequently if any abnormality is detected. Respiratory function is measured at each clinic appointment: usually every six months. Annual influenza vaccinations are advised.

Late ambulatory stage

As walking ability deteriorates, the use of a wheelchair (manual at first) will be considered. Therapy input is focused on maintaining movement and independence, although sometimes orthopaedic surgery may be needed to relieve tightness of joints. This will be considered appropriate only if John is still ambulant, and is usually restricted to releasing of the Achilles tendons. This would usually be avoided if splints are worn as part of a therapy regime, but John is not compliant in this respect. SCOPE (2016) offers advice to teachers on how to adapt teaching and learning activities as children's mobility changes. A closer watch is kept on the muscles of the heart and breathing, with additional echocardiogram surveillance, although no major changes would necessarily be expected yet. As soon as any changes are observed, then treatment with an angiotensin converting enzyme (ACE) inhibitor is started to reduce the blood pressure and the stress on the heart. A beta-blocker may be needed eventually to strengthen the heartbeat. Monitoring of weight and height in relation to steroid therapy will be continued, while muscle function and strength will also be measured at six-month intervals.

Early non-ambulatory stage

This is the phase in which the use of a wheelchair is unavoidable. It should be a pow-ered wheelchair to promote independence, though a manual wheelchair may be used at times or when access is restricted. Posture and movement receive special attention from physiotherapists, particularly of the shoulders, arms and hands. If upper limb function is becoming restricted due to weakness, then assessment may be arranged for equipment to promote independence of arm function. Once ambulation is lost trun-cal posture requires careful management, and assessment of the spine is necessary as scoliosis can develop. Problems with foot posture (foot drop) become common and can be uncomfortable or painful. Otherwise, monitoring of heart function continues, while decline of respiratory function is usual as a result of loss of the ability to walk. John is approaching this phase.

Late non-ambulatory stage

This is characterized by increasingly problematic upper limb function and body pos-ture. Additional efforts are needed to support independence through the provision of equipment and adaptive aids to normal daily activities and self-care. More fre-quent monitoring for heart and lung functioning is necessary with intervention as required.

4 **What psychological issues might arise? For a few minutes try to imagine being in John's place and think about how you might react to the news from the clinic.**

A In early childhood affected boys are unlikely to understand the progressive and fatal nature of the condition, and they are blind to the impacts that the disease will cause. They tend not to worry about these issues. Parents are advised to use clinic appoint-ments, meetings or other opportunities to start discussing the condition with the child in an age-appropriate manner. Parents are advised to be honest with their son and to start by explaining that he has a problem with his muscles. John is at an age where mobility is of huge importance. He wants to be able to do what his friends do, running around, climbing, jumping and generally being active. Yet now he has a dawning reali-zation that this is not to be and that his muscle weakness is getting worse. John also has to face further investigations regarding his heart function, and spinal fractures probably requiring treatment now or in the near future. It is a great burden for a 10 year old to carry.

When the need to use a wheelchair is introduced to younger children it might be accepted as a boost to mobility, but for John it represents further limitation and a dis-tinctive sign of being different and less able. He knows which secondary school he wants to attend and has been looking forward with the usual mix of excitement and trepidation to starting there after the summer holiday. Now, he may have to go in a wheelchair. Peer-group information and encouragement can be an effective prompt to re-evaluate such life challenges.

Extra resource

Watch the animated video created for and by teenage boys with DMD in the 'Takin' Charge' group of Action Duchenne (2015, https://www.youtube.com/watch?v=ClCFjRNjARY).

Resentment, fear, disappointment and helplessness are common reactions, and understandably so. Such responses may be manifest in different ways. There is often deep sadness, sometimes clinical depression and other times aggression. Challenging behaviour is common. The fact sheet for parents by the Muscular Dystrophy Campaign (2009) is particularly thorough and helpful. It is important that John's parents are accepting and supportive about the changes and challenges that he will face so that they can remain open and honest with him about his condition and what can be done to help him to stay well and independent. John will attend a mainstream school but will need an education healthcare plan to ensure that his needs are identified, supported and met. The aim is to promote his independence and maintain his self-esteem. An example of this is 'Active support': an approach that emphasizes participation and facilitation for pupils to achieve things for themselves rather than reliance on professionals. See the 'Well at School' website for an example of what schools might do to promote this (Chelsea Community Hospital School 2010).

THE OUTLOOK FOR JOHN

Duchenne muscular dystrophy is a serious, degenerative, muscle-wasting condition that is life limiting. Even with the best treatment, complications develop, particularly chest infections linked to reduced lung function and cardiac impairment leading to cardiac failure. Life expectancy has increased with better understanding of the condition and more effective treatment regimes. Although there is much variation between individual cases, currently, average life expectancy is to the late 20s and approaching 30 years (Muscular Dystrophy Association 2015). A study of patients in Germany established a median survival of 24 years, although patients who received overnight ventilation had a higher median survival of 27 years (Rall and Grim 2012). It is likely that further advances will increase this again.

This is all some way off in the future for John. He can expect to live an independent life with appropriate support, and many young men find their lives to be fulfilling. To achieve the most from life and to remain as healthy and able as possible will require proactive planning and a commitment to compliance with a medical management regime.

Activity

Finish this case by watching the inspiring video recorded by another John, aged 30: 'A Life Worth Living: Pushing the Limits of Duchenne' (Hastie 2012, https://www.youtube.com/watch?v=nrOOe_xXFa4).

> **Key points**
>
> - Duchenne muscular dystrophy is an X-linked degenerative condition that almost always affects boys. The condition is usually genetically inherited, but a non-inherited derivation from spontaneous gene mutation is also possible.
> - The condition progresses in predictable stages, with increasing muscle weakness, loss of ambulation and cardiorespiratory problems. There is no cure, but better treatments have resulted in longer life span.
> - Encouragement and promotion of continued independence are central aspects of intervention, together with psychological support. A fulfilling life of supported independence should be the aim.

REFERENCES

Action Duchenne (2015) (video). *Living with Duchenne Muscular Dystrophy (Video)*. London: Action Duchenne. Available at: https://www.youtube.com/watch?v=ClCFjRNjARY (accessed 26 January 2016).

Bushby K, Finkel R, Birnkrant D, et al. (2010a) Diagnosis and management of Duchenne muscular dystrophy, part 1: diagnosis, and pharmacological and psychosocial management. *The Lancet Neurology* 9 (1): 77–93 (DOI:10.1016/S1474-4422(09)70271-6). Available at: http://www.thelancet.com/journals/laneur/article/PIIS1474-4422(09)70271-6/fulltext (accessed 26 January 2016).

Bushby K, Finkel R, Birnkrant D, et al. (2010b) Diagnosis and management of Duchenne muscular dystrophy, part 2: implementation of multidisciplinary care. *The Lancet Neurology* 9(2): 177–189 (DOI: 10.1016/S1474-4422(09)70272-8). Available at: http://www.thelancet.com/journals/laneur/article/PIIS1474-4422(09)70272-8/fulltext (accessed 26 January 2016).

Chelsea Community Hospital School (2010) *Well at School*. London: CCHS. Available at: http://www.wellatschool.org/ (accessed 26 January 2016).

Duchenne Foundation Australia (2014) *The Duchenne Timeline (Video)*. Duchenne Foundation: Perth, Australia. Available at: https://www.youtube.com/watch?v=AF4D4TyE9NM (accessed 26 January 2016).

Hastie J (2012) *A Life Worth Living: Pushing the Limits of Duchenne*. Available at: https://www.youtube.com/watch?v=nr00e_xXFa4 (accessed 26 January 2016).

Muscular Dystrophy Association (2015) *Duchenne Muscular Dystrophy*. Chicago, IL: MDA. Available at: https://www.mda.org/disease/duchenne-muscular-dystrophy/overview (accessed 26 January 2016).

Muscular Dystrophy Campaign (2008) *Diagnosis and Treatment: Biopsies*. London: Muscular Dystrophy Campaign. Available at: http://www.muscular-dystrophy.org/assets/0002/2946/Muscle_biopsies.pdf (accessed 26 January 2016).

Muscular Dystrophy Campaign (2009) *Family, Relationships and Emotional Issues: Behavioural Issues in DMD*. London: Muscular Dystrophy Campaign. Available at: http://www.muscular-dystrophy.org/assets/0002/3001/Behavioural_issues.pdf (accessed 26 January 2016).

North Star Clinical Network (2014) *North Star Ambulatory Assessment*. London: Muscular Dystrophy Campaign. Available at: http://www.muscular-dystrophy.org/assets/0000/6388/NorthStar.pdf (accessed 26 January 2016).

Rall S, Grimm T (2012) Survival in Duchenne muscular dystrophy. *Acta Myologica* 31(2): 117–120. Available at: http://www.ncbi.nlm.nih.gov/pmc/articles/PMC3476855/ (accessed 26 January 2016).

SCOPE (2016) *Impairments and Conditions*. London: SCOPE. Available at: http://www.scope.org.uk/support/professionals/learning-together/impairment-conditions-1 (accessed 10 Feburary 2016).

Treat-NMD (2011) *The Diagnosis and Management of Duchenne Muscular Dystrophy: A Guide for Families*. Newcastle: Treat-NMD. Available at: http://www.treat-nmd.eu/care/dmd/diagnosis-management-DMD/ (accessed 26 January 2016).

Osteosarcoma in a teenager who develops secondaries

Tony Long and Andrea Stevenson

Case outline

Emily, who is 13 years old, is an academically capable teenager who is keen on sport and plays for her school team, has been complaining of knee and lower leg pain for a few weeks. Initially, her parents believed this to be the result of an old injury during netball practice. She had been to the general practitioner (GP) several times, and the GP, finding no obvious cause on examination, diagnosed a sprain injury and prescribed rest and analgesic.

The pain intensified with little relief, disrupting sleep. Finally, her parents took Emily to the local accident and emergency department (A&E) where x-ray confirmed a mass within the bone of the tibia. The staff contacted the oncology department, and a specialist orthopaedic consultation was arranged. This led to biopsy under anaesthetic, and a week later the diagnosis of osteosarcoma was established. At a tertiary referral centre, a treatment regime was devised of chemotherapy to be followed by surgery, and, depending upon the findings during surgery, further chemotherapy.

OSTEOSARCOMA

Osteosarcoma is a malignant cancer that forms in bone, usually in the arms or legs (especially near the knee) (Figure 22.1). It is rare in young children and more common in middle childhood and teenagers. The ends of long bones, where growth occurs, are common sites for the tumour to commence. These sites are especially active during puberty, resulting in the higher incidence in children at that time of life. The cause is not known, and trauma is not a contributing factor.

Extra resource

Browse the Radiopaedia site to see more radiographic images of cases of osteosarcoma (2015, http://radiopaedia.org/articles/osteosarcoma).

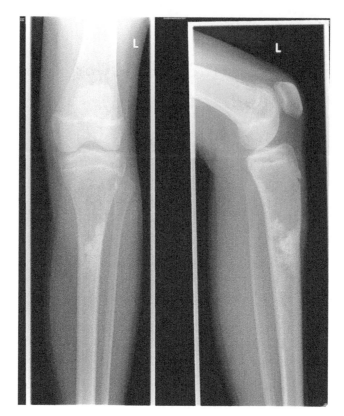

Figure 22.1 Anterior and lateral x-ray views of osteosarcoma in the tibia

The presenting symptoms are normally intensifying pain with swelling at the site. Diagnosis is by x-ray and scan, confirmed by biopsy and blood tests. Treatment varies according to the position and stage of the tumour, but normally involves chemotherapy to shrink the tumour, followed by surgery (amputation or removal of the affected bone – usually replaced by a prosthesis). Most children are cured, but delay in diagnosis and the site of the tumour can result in a poor outcome.

1   **Try to put yourself in Emily's position and think about her possible responses to this devastating news. Consider that she will spend long periods feeling ill, still immobile following the surgery, with repeated stays in hospital, removed from her peer group and with her plans for life all in question.**

A   You probably thought about both physical and psychological effects: the impact on her self-image, the gruelling nature and side effects of treatment, the termination of growing independence, and the anxiety caused by fear of a poor prognosis. A wonderful account is provided for other young people with cancer by Megan Blunt (then aged 14) of her experience as a patient (Blunt 2013).

SELF-IMAGE AND PSYCHOLOGICAL IMPACT

For a teenage girl, you would expect that physical appearance would be important, as would maintaining a place within a peer network. These are likely to pose problems since Emily will be separated from her friends during treatment, missing school for a full year or more, and because of hair loss and nausea during chemotherapy. Cancer remains a difficult topic for most people to discuss, and this may isolate Emily emotionally from those about whom she cares.

Emotional regression is common, in which teenagers revert to an earlier stage of development, becoming dependent again physically, psychologically and emotionally on parents or carers. This is prompted by physical inability to continue as before and by the enormity of the psychological challenge posed by the diagnosis. Clearly, this has an impact on how nurses will approach discussions and decision-making with Emily.

PHYSICAL ILL HEALTH

Nausea and vomiting, diarrhoea or constipation, tiredness, and sore mouth are common side effects of chemotherapy. A typical protocol would be Doxorubicin, Cisplatin and Methotrexate for 10 weeks before surgery, then again for 18 weeks afterwords: a gruelling regime.

> Almost a year after the initial diagnosis, repeat x-ray and computed tomography scan of the chest showed evidence of metastatic disease (secondary spread). A right-sided thoracotomy was undertaken to remove affected tissue, and additional chemotherapy was instituted. The most recent scan shows further metastases on the left side, so a second thoracotomy is planned, to be followed by further chemotherapy.

Although most children are cured, there is always an anxious wait to learn the result of subsequent scans in case it is found that the tumour has spread to other regions (usually the lungs). Some 20–25 per cent of patients with osteosarcoma present with already detectable metastatic disease (National Cancer Institute 2014), but up to 80 per cent of patients with high grade osteosarcoma may already have metastases that do not show on imaging tests at first diagnosis. This is clearly what Emily and her parents have been dreading, and it indicates a poor prognosis (a forecast of the likely course of a disease). Emily will already have seen friends that she has made on the oncology unit die, and it is likely that she will already be questioning the possibility of her own death.

The prognosis will be discussed with Emily and her parents at the earliest opportunity once the medical case is clear. However, reactions to this can vary. Some teenagers may refuse to accept this, holding to the belief all through the palliative care phase that they will be cured. Others choose to make the most of the time left to them in active pursuit of the achievement of desired goals. The importance of both physical and psychological support for patients at this point is stressed by SIOPE (2009).

2 **Think for a few minutes: how would you break this news to Emily if it were your responsibility? As a student nurse this would not be your role, of course, but the skills of breaking bad or sad news are a vital component of nursing. You may be on duty, caring for Emily after she has received bad news, and need to think of ways to communicate effectively with her. Think of the reassurance that is needed as well as her emotional needs.**

A Reflect now on the assumptions that you made: about the nature and depth of the information to be conveyed; the possible responses; how to ensure that the information and its implications have been taken in; and what needs to follow the disclosure to ensure that the patient and family are adequately supported. You might even have thought about how to look after your own needs after undertaking this challenging task. See the guidance from the Royal College of Nursing (2012).

The nursing team must move now to predict the problems that Emily will face as her treatment continues. These are likely to be many and sometimes severe. Much of the difficulty will result from the side effects of prolonged chemotherapy.

3 **What is chemotherapy and what effects does it have on the body?**

A Chemotherapy is a treatment modality that employs cytotoxic drugs to shrink the tumour and to kill cancer cells outside the main tumour mass. Differing cytotoxic drugs interfere with various elements of the cell division process. Since they exert the greatest effect on rapidly dividing cells, they are especially effective in destroying tumour cells. However, rapidly dividing cells are found in other sites in the body, especially in the bone marrow, in the lining of the digestive tract and in hair follicles. This leads to the side effects detailed in Figure 22.2 and discussed below.

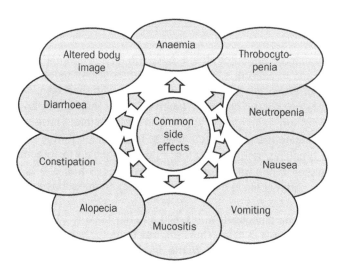

Figure 22.2 Side effects of chemotherapy

SIDE EFFECTS OF CHEMOTHERAPY

Anaemia

This occurs because of a reduced number of circulating red blood cells. It may be recognized clinically by pallor, lethargy, breathlessness, headaches or fainting. Careful monitoring of blood test results will prompt the need for transfusion if the haemoglobin falls below 80 g/dl.

Thrombocytopenia

This refers to a reduced number of platelets in the blood, leaving a patient prone to uncontrolled bleeding. As with other problems with the blood count, there are protocols to guide intervention. The treatment is a transfusion of platelets. Normal platelet count is measured as more than 150 thousand platelets per microlitre of plasma. If this falls below 20 thousand, transfusion will be instigated (Table 22.1). Emily will bruise easily at a count below 50 thousand, and the count needs to be above 75 thousand for chemotherapy to be administered.

Neutropenia

This refers to the lack of neutrophil cells, which are the most common white blood cells. They destroy foreign micro-organisms through release of antimicrobial proteins (degranulation) and engulfing bacteria (phagocytosis), and they also recruit additional white cells to the site of inflammation and infection. Neutrophils are largely responsible for the formation of pus. A neutrophil count of less than $1.0 \times 10^9/l$ (that is: less than 1000 million per litre of blood) leads to the patient being immunocompromised (unable to react effectively to infections). This is neutropenia. Regular monitoring of body temperature is vital. If one recording is above 38.5°C or if the temperature is above 38°C twice in one hour, then blood is taken for culture and antibiotic treatment is started.

Nausea and vomiting

Cytotoxic drugs cause sickness, which is managed with anti-emetics. Usually this is in the form of ondansetron given orally or intravenously every eight hours by the nurse.

Table 22.1 Indicators for platelet transfusion

Platelet count	Additional factors
Below 20	(Especially if febrile)
Below 30	Having a lumber puncture
Below 40	Newly diagnosed brain tumour

Additional action is possible if this is ineffective as observed by the nurse. This may be metoclopramide (Maxalon), and sometimes dexamethasone is used in combination with metoclopramide. The intensity of the nausea can be anticipated so that sometimes patients can feel sick or vomit even on entering the unit for their treatment. Lorazepam is sometimes prescribed, to be taken the night before chemotherapy is given, in order to control these symptoms.

(Oral) mucositis

Mucosal cells (which divide rapidly), in this case in the mouth, are affected by cytotoxic drugs. This is painful, and causes dry mouth, ulceration, difficulty in swallowing and problems in the gastrointestinal tract. Effective oral hygiene and relief of pain are the main interventions. Nurses may be advised in this care by the guidelines from the *United Kingdom Children's Cancer Study Group – Paediatric Oncology Nurses Forum* (2006). However, the pain and discomfort can be so severe as to require feeding by tube, while infection of the ulcerated mouth may lead to septicaemia.

Alopecia

Hair loss also results from chemotherapy. The pattern varies greatly from thinning to complete hair loss (including eyebrows and lashes). Indeed, it is important to make teenagers aware that all hair on the body could be lost depending upon the chemotherapy regime. Hats and caps are recommended, while real hair wigs can be provided. Psychological support is an important nursing intervention since alopecia can be intensely distressing for some patients.

Diarrhoea and constipation

Gastrointestinal disturbances are very common and result from the lining of the gut being damaged by cytotoxic agents. Laxatives are used routinely, and soreness round the anus can be soothed with creams and pain relief. Anal fissures are not uncommon, and sensitive assessments are required in oncology patients as they can cause infections that break down the mucus membranes.

4 **What are the ongoing care needs for Emily?**

A As time goes on and control of the metastases is lost the outcome becomes overtly uncertain. Emily and her family may struggle to look towards a future. They will need help to find courage and confidence, and to plan in order to impose some kind of control over the unpredictable situation in which they find themselves. Prediction of symptoms is only available for known disease, and an advanced package of care can then begin to be collated and shared with Emily and parents. It is important at this stage to involve the multidisciplinary team in hospital – and at home if this is where Emily chooses to stay. Regular meetings are needed throughout this period, to maintain symptom management.

CACHEXIA

Chronic malnutrition resulting from poor appetite, gastrointestinal problems, and effects of pain-controlling medications results in weight loss and gradual degradation. The emaciation of cachexia makes the skin prone to pressure sores. Maximizing Emily's caloric intake is important, as is standard pressure-area care as her mobility decreases. Emily will have choices about supplemental feeding, whether the use of nasogastric feeds or calorific milkshakes. For many teenagers like Emily, 'shots' of drinks containing 200 calories are popular. Observation of skin integrity is important so as to protect vulnerable tissue areas and promote comfort.

HICKMAN LINE

This central venous catheter, which will have been inserted at the beginning of treatment, will require flushing weekly when not in use to maintain patency. Central line access can be used for pain and symptom management at any time throughout the trajectory of care.

PAIN RELIEF

Once paracetamol becomes ineffective in controlling pain, oral morphine (Oromorph and MST [sustained release morphine]) will be used to keep Emily free from pain. (Ibuprofen is not used for patients undergoing chemotherapy since it tends to deplete the platelets.)

5 **Discuss the role of other types of therapy**

Ⓐ **PHYSIOTHERAPY**

Emily will have a confirmed relationship with the physiotherapist from diagnosis throughout her treatment, aiding mobility safely before surgery, and implementing rehabilitation after surgery. On discharge home, Emily will have returned to the hospital for continued intensive physiotherapy. As changes to mobility status occur the physiotherapist can aid Emily in adaptations to help her feel safe, and this will be in conjunction with the community occupational therapist.

OCCUPATIONAL THERAPY

The community occupational therapist has a vital role in assessing Emily and her home for suitable equipment to aid her independence. This can also give an indication of how Emily is coping with the changes to her body, as the necessity of equipment for managing normal daily activities can be difficult for teenagers to accept.

Activity

Complete the case by taking a little time to read the Macmillan Cancer Support (2012) leaflet for young people 'I'm still me' to see the importance of thinking about young people with cancer as having emotional and psychological needs as well as physical needs. Notice the concerns that they might have and how a positive, measured, factual response is made to these.

Key points

- Osteosarcoma (and other cancers in childhood) are often not diagnosed as soon as they might be, but early diagnosis is linked to better outcomes. Most children are cured, but some tumours are diagnosed too late or are sited such as to lead to a poor prognosis.
- The medical team is honest with children and parents about risk factors and possible outcomes. Waiting for a diagnosis, test and scan results, and potentially bad news can be consuming for parents. They must be able to count on the nurse for support.
- Much skilled nursing care is needed to address the multiple and often severe side effects of treatment. This will focus on physical, psychological and emotional needs.

REFERENCES

Blunt M (2013) *Chemotherapy, Cakes And Cancer. (An A to Z Guide to Living with Childhood Cancer)*. London: CLIC Sargent. Available at: http://www.clicsargent.org.uk/sites/files/clicsargent/field/field_document/Chemotherapy%2C%20Cakes%20and%20Cancer%202013%20update.PDF (accessed 10 February 2016).

Macmillan Cancer Support (2012) *I'm Still Me – A Guide for Young People Living with Cancer*. London: Macmillan Cancer Support. Available at: http://www.macmillan.org.uk/Documents/Cancerinfo/Imstillme.pdf (accessed 27 January 2016).

National Cancer Intitute (2014) *Osteosarcoma and MFH of Bone with Metastatic Disease at Diagnosis. Bethseda*, MD: NCI. Available at: http://www.cancer.gov/cancertopics/pdq/treatment/osteosarcoma/HealthProfessional/page6 (accessed 27 January 2016).

Royal College of Nursing (2012) *RCN Competences: Palliative Care for Children and Young People*. London: RCN. Available at: https://www2.rcn.org.uk/__data/assets/pdf_file/0012/488991/004_328.pdf (accessed 10 February 2016).

SIOPE (The European Society of Paediatric Oncology) (2009) *European Standards of Care for Children with Cancer*. Warsaw: SIOPE. Available at: http://www.siope.eu/wp-content/uploads/2013/09/European_Standards_final_2011.pdf (accessed 10 February 2016).

United Kingdom Children's Cancer Study Group – Paediatric Oncology Nurses Forum (2006) *Mouth Care for Children and Young People with Cancer: Evidence-based Guidelines. Guideline Report Version 1.0.* Manchester: UKCCSG-PONF. Available at: http://www.rcpch.ac.uk/sites/default/ files/asset_library/Research/Clinical%20Effectiveness/Endorsed%20guidelines/Mouth%20 Care%20for%20CYP%20with%20cancer%20(cancer%20study%20group/mouth_care_cyp_ cancer_guidelinev2.pdf (accessed 10 February 2016).

Transition to adult services: cystic fibrosis

Leyonie Higgins and Janet Edgar

Case outline

Sabrina is now 14 years old. She was diagnosed shortly after birth with meconium ileus, a condition that causes the gut to become blocked with meconium: a thick, dark, sticky substance that is made in all babies' intestines before being born. Sabrina required urgent surgery to relieve the meconium blockage.

As Sabrina was born before 2007 she was not screened for cystic fibrosis shortly after birth using the newborn blood spot screening programme, which tests for the most common mutations of the gene that causes cystic fibrosis. As a baby, Sabrina's father noticed that when he kissed Sabrina her skin tasted salty. Sabrina was diagnosed following her surgery by a sweat test.

This case will explore issues around Sabrina's transition to adult services.

THE SWEAT TEST

A sweat test measures the amount of salt in sweat. It is usually done by applying a very weak and painless electric current to a small area of skin to which a harmless chemical has been applied, which causes that area of skin to sweat. A sample of the sweat is then collected and analysed. If the salt content in the sweat is abnormally high, this confirms cystic fibrosis.

1 **What are the predominant internal organs that are affected by cystic fibrosis?**

(a) **All of them.**
(b) **The lungs and digestive system.**
(c) **Kidney and spleen.**

A The correct answer is (b). Cystic fibrosis is one of the UK's most common life-threatening inherited diseases. Cystic fibrosis is caused by a single defective gene. As a result, the internal organs, especially the lungs and digestive system, become clogged with thick sticky mucus resulting in chronic infections and inflammation in the lungs and difficulty digesting food.

2 **How did Sabrina get cystic fibrosis?**

(a) She caught it from a virus or bacteria.
(b) It developed in the womb.
(c) It is a genetic condition.

A The correct answer is (c). Cystic fibrosis is a genetic condition. In the UK, 1 person in 25 carries the faulty cystic fibrosis gene usually without knowing. If two carriers have a baby, the child has a one in four chance of having cystic fibrosis. (see Cases 20 on Sickle cell disease and 21 on Duchenne muscular dystrophy.)

3 **What symptoms will Sabrina experience because of her cystic fibrosis?**

(a) Aching joints.
(b) Cough, wheezing, shortness of breath and breathing difficulties, and repeated chest infections.
(c) Bloated abdomen and tummy aches, constipation and prolonged diarrhoea.
(d) All of the above.

A The correct answer is (d). In people with cystic fibrosis the lungs make thicker sputum (mucus) than normal, which can trap bacteria in the small airways and lead to infection. Thickened mucus secretions block the normal flow of digestive juices from the pancreas, which means food cannot be digested or absorbed properly, in particular fatty foods and fat-soluble vitamins (vitamins A, D, E and K), which can cause malnutrition leading to poor growth and poor weight gain. Other symptoms can include sinus infections and nasal polyps. Some children and adults with cystic fibrosis may also get cystic fibrosis related diabetes, arthritis, osteoporosis and liver problems. The severity of symptoms can vary and not all people with cystic fibrosis will have every symptom. You can read more about how problems with cystic fibrosis come about in an article by Bowen and Hull (2015).

4 **How will Sabrina's cystic fibrosis be treated?**

(a) Heart medications + salbutamol + physiotherapy.
(b) Lactulose + Becotide + physiotherapy.
(c) Physiotherapy + antibiotics + enzymes and vitamins.
(d) Surgery + heart medications + physiotherapy.

A The correct answer is (c). Sabrina will have to undergo a rigorous daily regime of treatments to stay healthy, which will include taking antibiotics and inhaled drugs to clear mucus and fight infections, taking dozens of enzyme pills to digest food and having physiotherapy morning and night. See how this is presented to families by the Cystic Fibrosis Trust (2015a).

Sabrina is in the last two years of her secondary school education and is starting preparations for her final exams. She has just started her menstrual periods, although these are irregular. As a student nurse it would not be your responsibility to initiate the following discussions; however you might be engaged in conversations with Sabrina, her father and their nurse specialist. You will need to consider that cystic fibrosis can be a very isolating disease as people with cystic fibrosis cannot mix because of the risk of cross infection.

Activity

Reflect on how this isolation might affect a teenager; the effects of hormones during adolescence and how these two issues might affect compliance with treatment and school regimes and Sabrina's thoughts for her future.

5 **Sabrina is starting to question if it is worth her doing any work for her exams as she has cystic fibrosis, what advice would you give her?**

A Children with cystic fibrosis are as academically able as their peers; Sabrina needs to be made aware that examination boards can make certain allowances for pupils with cystic fibrosis. Additional time can be allowed (normally up to 25 per cent) for all types of examination. If necessary a candidate with cystic fibrosis can be given treatment during a supervised break. Alternatively, subject to approval from the exam board, arrangements can be made for Sabrina to take exams outside her schools exam centre (at home or in hospital).

Great steps forward in specialist care and treatment have meant that people with cystic fibrosis are living longer and healthier lives, but many will reach a point where they require a lung or liver transplant to prolong their life. Sabrina needs to be encouraged to discuss her plans and goals for her future. She may need to be encouraged to consider a career that reduces cross-infection risks.

6 **What would you explain to Sabrina about her fertility given that her menstrual cycle is irregular?**

A Bray et al. (2010) found that health professionals varied in their approach and competence in initiating and engaging in conversations with young people about sexual health and relationships. Lack of knowledge was a particularly impeding factor in the professional's ability to undertake this part of their role. They tended to focus on physiology, fertility and medication, but often failed to discuss issues of relationships and sexuality.

7 **What approach would you take, and what aspects of the issue might make you feel uncomfortable or less competent?**

A Women with cystic fibrosis may find that their menstrual cycle becomes absent or irregular if they are underweight; there is also an increased thickness of cervical mucus, which can sometimes reduce fertility. However, some women with cystic fibrosis can have a successful pregnancy, though it may take longer than usual before conceiving a baby. Sabrina should also be given the same sexual health information as any other teenager, however, careful thought is needed about types of contraception because of the regular use of additional antibiotics. It is important to include discussion of sexual relationships as well as physiological matters.

At Sabrina's next clinic appointment her named nurse discusses with Sabrina and her father that at their next and subsequent appointments they will start to talk about Sabrina's transition to the regional adult cystic fibrosis services. This is discussed initially from the age of 13 but in more depth from 15 years.

---

8   **How would you help to prepare Sabrina's father for Sabrina's transition to the adult services?**

A   Sabrina's father has been her main carer and been involved in all aspects of her care since birth. As children grow they need to be encouraged to become independent and take responsibility for themselves; Sabrina should be treated no differently. Sabrina's father may need some encouragement and support to relinquish his roles and encourage Sabrina to take responsibility for decisions regarding her cares and treatment. Sabrina's father will need to begin to take on a more supportive role. The beginnings of this transfer of roles and responsibilities from the father to Sabrina can often be a difficult and emotional time for everyone, but advice and support are available (Department of Health 2006).

9   **How would you help prepare Sabrina for her transition to the adult cystic fibrosis service?**

A   Take some time to review the work of National Voices (2015) and what children and young people themselves have said about their expectations of coordinated services – 'The I Statements'. The National Network of Parent Carers Forum (2015) summarizes this as follows.

- When I use a new service, my care plan is known in advance and respected.
- When I move between services or settings, there is a plan in place for what happens next.
- I know in advance where I am going, what I will be provided with, and who will be my main point of professional contact.
- I am given information about any medicines I take with me – their purpose, how to take them, potential side effects.
- If I still need contact with previous services/professionals, this is made possible.

Consider that Sabrina and her father have been coming to the same hospital; having the same routines and seeing the same staff for many years. It is therefore important that the idea of transfer to adult services is introduced at an appropriate time for Sabrina. The transition period will take a few years; it will involve lots of consultations between Sabrina, her current specialist cystic fibrosis centre, her father and clinicians at the adult centre to make the move as easy as possible. UK services transfer teenagers to adult cystic fibrosis services between the ages of 16 and 18 years.

Change of any kind can be daunting, but some people can also find it an exciting prospect. It is therefore important to discuss with Sabrina how she feels about her impending transfer to help identify and deal with any anxieties. This is especially important as she may also be transferring from high school to college. The Cystic Fibrosis Trust (2015b) provides advice and information for families about transition. Sabrina's current team will provide a plan for Sabrina and her father about what the transition involves, including the date of her final paediatric clinic or admission before moving on to the adult centre. Sabrina will also receive a 'transition document' containing information about the centre to which she will be transferring. The Care Quality Commission (2014), having found deficiencies in transition planning to be widespread, has provided guidance based on feedback from young people who have experienced transition.

- Commissioners must listen to and learn from young people and their families.
- Existing good practice guidance must be followed to ensure young people are properly supported through transition.
- General practitioners should be more involved, at an earlier stage, in planning for transition.
- Adolescence/young adulthood should be recognized across the health service as an important developmental phase – with NHS England and Health Education England taking a leadership role.

Some centres in the UK do a joint transition clinic and the teenager is seen with both the paediatric team and the adult team in the same clinic so the teenager can get to know the adult team, and the paediatric team can discuss their care and treatment with the adult team. However, this can be intimidating as this may lead to a room full of professionals – two doctors, two physiotherapists, two nurses and two dieticians.

In Manchester the service has moved away from this following feedback from families. Initially, the parents will have been invited to a joint event with both teams to discuss the adult service. In the run up to the transfer a visit is done at home with the teenager's paediatric nurse, a nurse from the adult team and an adult social worker. This allows an informal approach to discuss the service, and allows the family to ask questions. The family is also offered a visit to the adult hospital.

The Care Quality Commission (2014) also found examples of services and processes that had worked well for young people in transition, and these messages should be a guide to what Sabrina should expect.

- Having consistent staff members who knew about the conditions and the young person's history.
- Providing adolescent clinics.
- Good communication with young people, their parents and each other.
- Providing good information about what to expect.

Key points

- Cystic fibrosis is a common, life-threatening, inherited disease in which thick, sticky mucus clogs the internal organs, particularly the lungs and digestive system, causing recurrent or chronic infection and problems with digestion.

- Despite a grinding regime of daily treatments, children and young people who are affected can aspire to normal school achievement, although social life is adversely affected by periods of illness, the need to avoid infection and daily routines.
- Those with cystic fibrosis should experience planned, coordinated transition to adult services, and helpful guidelines are provided for this – both in structure and in approach. Managing the change in roles of parents and children requires tact, insight and patience, so transition will normally occur over a few years.

REFERENCES

Bowen S-J, Hull J (2015) The basic science of cystic fibrosis. *Paediatrics and Child Health* 25(4): 159–164.

Bray L, McKenna J, Sanders C, Pritchard E (2010) Discussing sexual and relationship health with young people in an acute children's hospital. *Journal of Research in Nursing* 17(3): 231–241.

Care Quality Commission (2014) *From the Pond into the Sea: Children's Transition to Adult Services.* Newcastle: CQC. Available at: https://www.cqc.org.uk/sites/default/files/CQC_Transition%20 Report.pdf (accessed 27 January 2016).

Cystic Fibrosis Trust (2015a) *Living with Cystic Fibrosis.* London: Cystic Fibrosis Trust. Available at: http://www.cysticfibrosis.org.uk/about-cf/living-with-cystic-fibrosis (accessed 27 January 2016).

Cystic Fibrosis Trust (2015b) *Transition.* London: Cystic Fibrosis Trust. Available at: http://www.cysticfibrosis.org.uk/about-cf/living-with-cystic-fibrosis/transition (accessed 27 January 2016).

Department of Health (2006) *Transition: Getting It Right for Young People.* London: DH. Available at: http://webarchive.nationalarchives.gov.uk/20130107105354/http:/www.dh.gov.uk/prod_consum_dh/groups/dh_digitalassets/@dh/@en/documents/digitalasset/dh_4132149.pdf (accessed 27 January 2016).

National Network of Parent Carers Forum (2015) *What Good Integrated Care Looks Like.* London: NNCPF. Available at: http://www.nnpcf.org.uk/what-good-integrated-care-looks-like-in-transition/ (accessed 27 January 2016).

National Voices (2015) *My Life, My Support, My Choice.* London: National Voices. Available at: http://www.nationalvoices.org.uk/sites/www.nationalvoices.org.uk/files/tlapmylifemysupportmychoice_final.pdf (accessed 27 January 2016).

Index

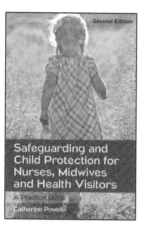

Safeguarding and Child Protection for Nurses, Midwives and Health Visitors
A Practical Guide

Powell

ISBN: 9780335262526 (Paperback)
eISBN: 9780335262533

2015

Nurses, midwives and health visitors have a statutory duty to safeguard and promote the welfare of children and young people. In this clear and invaluable guide, Catherine Powell focuses on the practical aspects of safeguarding and how healthcare professionals should respond to safeguarding children concerns.

Key features of the book include:

- Setting out the roles and responsibilities of nurses, midwives and health visitors working in a range of settings, including those working primarily with adult clients
- Realistic case scenarios of physical, emotional and sexual abuse and neglect, covering infants, toddlers, school-age children and adolescents
- Explanations of inter-agency working and the roles of other key players such as children's social care, the police and education services
- 'Markers of Good Practice' boxes highlighting lessons for practice

www.mheducation.co.uk

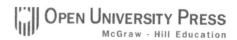

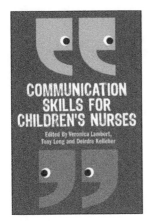

Communication Skills for Children's Nurses

Lambert

ISBN: 9780335242863 (Paperback)
eISBN: 9780335242887

2012

This guide will help children's nurses communicate with confidence, sensitivity and effectiveness, to meet the individual needs of children and their families. The book explores different aspects of communicating in this challenging environment using vignettes, examples, practice insights and tips.

The book emphasises the importance of listening to and respecting children's views and rights, in addition to respecting parent responsibility, rights and duty to act in the child's best interests. The authors show how a balance between protective exclusion and facilitated inclusion is core to communicating with children and families.

Key topics covered include:

- Communicating during challenging and sensitive times
- The importance of being culturally sensitive and self-aware
- Meeting the needs of vulnerable and disadvantaged children
- Engaging with children who experience difficulty in communicating
- Ethical and legal dimensions of communicating with families
- Appreciating the nature of 'voice' in research with children

www.mheducation.co.uk

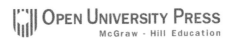

OPEN UNIVERSITY PRESS
McGraw - Hill Education

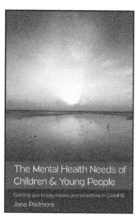

The Mental Health Needs of Children and Young People
Guiding you to key issues and practices in CAMHS

Padmore

ISBN: 9780335263905 (Paperback)
eBook: 9780335263912
2015

This book is an accessible and practical guide to all of the key issues and practices in mental health care for children and young people, aimed at all health and social care professionals working with this age group and partner agencies who work alongside child and adolescent mental health services.

Written by an expert in the field, the book brings clarity to practice by exploring and explaining the context, role and processes involving child and adolescent mental health services. It also sets out the specific mental health difficulties young people and their families present to services as well as how to make good health assessments, plans and interventions used in the treatment of children and young people – including managing risk and safeguarding.

Key features include:

Questions to encourage your reflection on different key issues in your own practice
Up-to-date information on current policy
Key points summaries and suggested further reading at the end of each chapter

www.mheducation.co.uk

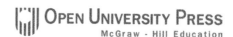
OPEN UNIVERSITY PRESS
McGraw - Hill Education